Eat Your Way to Health

The simply delicious way to feel better,
look younger and reach your ideal weight

Includes over 100 recipes!

by

Kaaren Jordan
&
Crit Taylor

HealingEssences.com
(805) 245-9908

This book is dedicated to Eileen Poole who through her unique gift carried on the amazing work of Dr. Henry Bieler in her own way. Eileen opened me to a new path many years ago, and her continuing guidance supports me still.

During one of our early sessions, Eileen encouraged me to study the traditional healing art of Jin Shin Jyutsu®. As a client of Eileen's, it was my experience of Dr. Bieler's wisdom through her life changing work that inspired me to also study nutrition. I will be forever grateful to Eileen for planting the seeds for what is now my life's work and passion.

I also want to give special thanks for the invaluable support of all my wonderful clients and friends during the creation of this book.

And finally I am especially grateful to my husband, whose hard work, patience, love and faith in me has kept me on track through some very rough roads.

Kaaren Jordan

Every effort has been made by the authors of this book to provide accurate information. However, due to the law, we the authors cannot and do not make any explicit claims for nutrient efficacy, or the treatment, mitigation, prevention or cure of disease. If you are ill we recommend that you see a qualified medical professional. The authors also disclaim any responsibility for losses or damages that may occur from use of information in this book.

Table of Contents

1 Food & Your Immune System — 1

2 Diet/Low Fat Products Can Cause Problems — 4

3 Food Sensitivities — 6

4 What to Eat & What Not to Eat — 8

5 Other Toxins To Avoid — 23

6 Psychological & Emotional Factors — 27

7 Exercise & Other Self Healing Techniques — 31

8 The Daily Body Feedback Journal — 32

9 Simply Delicious Recipes — 35

- Cereal and Grain Dishes — 37
- Entrees — 42
- Soups — 53
- Salads — 60
- Vegetables — 62
- Sauces/Spreads/Dips/Dressing — 67
- Fruits and Desserts — 73

10 Sample Menus — 80

11 Falling Off The Wagon — 82

12 Putting It All Together — 83

Food & Your Immune System

Around 500 B.C. Hippocrates, the father of Western medicine, imparted to his students the most basic and profound medical truth, "Thy food shall be thy remedy." Inspired by this idea, in the late 1920's a young Henry Bieler M.D. devoted his life to using foods as medicine. Then during the next 50 years he proceeded to cure thousands of seriously ill patients relying solely on foods for treatment. The information in this book is primarily based on my understanding of Dr. Bieler's work combined with information from my studies and experiences.

A toxic body is the root cause of disease

Dr. Bieler disagreed with most of his medical colleagues when he declared that germs and viruses were not the cause of disease. He said that germs and viruses are present and multiply readily in a toxic body, but it is the toxemia and not the germs/viruses that is the root cause of disease. He felt the most effective way to regain permanent health was to reduce the toxemia through proper foods, and thus enable the body's immune system to control the germs and viruses.

What causes a toxic body?

Dr. Bieler discovered that the main cause of most people's toxemia was their life-style choices, ie. primarily their eating habits. A wide variety of recent long term studies, including the U.S. Department of Health and Human Services 1991 *Healthy People 2000* report, has largely validated Dr. Bieler's opinion by concluding that roughly 75% of all disease is caused by life-style choices. We also have found from our own observations that a person's emotional / mental state is a significant contributing factor.

The cure for a toxic body

Dr. Bieler felt that low starch vegetables should be the main food group in most diets. This is partly because low starch vegetables greatly help support the organs of elimination in their cleansing processes. Dr. Bieler discovered that most people's poor dietary habits made their bodies highly acidic. And since low starch vegetables are more alkaline than starchy vegetables or grains, they serve to balance the body's PH. This is very important since a significant PH imbalance depresses the immune system and has a negative effect on all body systems.

Natural Supplements

With 21st century hectic lifestyles, food choices and nutrient deficiencies in the soil our food is grown in, most of us need additional amounts of vitamins and minerals to stay healthy. Even though "natural" supplements are derived from natural sources, they are highly concentrated and processed. I feel it is best to view this category as "supplements to" rather than "substitutes for" a healthy diet and lifestyle. My preference is powders and liquids first and capsules second since there are usually less binders and fillers than are found in tablets.

Natural supplements . . . less is best

Nutritional supplements unfortunately can have drawbacks. Many supplements are not readily bio-available, meaning that your body has to do a lot of work to digest and assimilate them. High amounts or inappropriate types put a strain on the liver and kidneys by making them work overtime. I generally recommend additional vitamin D, E, C and an omega and multi mineral formulated for your sex, age and activity levels. In some cases selected additional supplements may be beneficial, but that is on a purely individual basis.

How does stress help create a toxic body?

It is generally accepted that overall accumulated stress is very unhealthful, especially for your immune system. Chronic stress can produce a wide variety of unwanted reactions, including making your body more acidic. When you add this to a diet that also helps create an acidic PH, you can see that something needs to be done to restore balance. Otherwise illness and disease will eventually occur. Fortunately you can learn to achieve and maintain a healthy balance through the easy practices outlined in this book.

The wise use of drugs

Although Dr. Bieler successfully treated the vast majority of his patients with food instead of drugs, this does not mean that you should simply drop all medications and only follow the guidelines in this book. Quite the contrary, I strongly urge you to work ongoing with qualified medical professionals in your healing process. Dr. Bieler's chief complaint, that modern doctors seem to have lost sight of the fact that foods may be the most effective way to treat most illnesses, should be considered. Drugs, he correctly noted, often have side effects that further degrade the overall health of the patient. Also he felt that most drugs were only treating surface issues instead of dealing with the root cause, namely the patient's toxemia. So with this in mind I urge you to find a balance that works for you.

Proper foods help no matter what else you do

The great thing about using foods as a healing tool, is that they work by themselves or in conjunction with anything else that you are doing. It does not matter, whether you are going through chemotherapy or you regularly do yoga, eating the appropriate foods for your unique system makes a difference. And since we all have to eat, it makes sense to me that we might as well use foods to our advantage. The way I see it our food either nourishes and heals us or it is a foreign substance that our body struggles to deal with.

The information in this book can help your immune system directly and indirectly

Simply put, the guidelines in this book are designed to help you discover what works best for you. Everybody is different so it is impossible to design just one diet that will suit everybody. However Dr. Bieler and those that have followed him noted a number of general guidelines that held true for most people; and so we present that information here as a substantial foundation on which you can build.

Some of the things presented here may provide immediate and noticeable effect. Many people begin to feel the positive effects of the Bieler's Broth and or low starch vegetables right away. This is because their bodies are starved for the unique and irreplaceable qualities these foods embody. Another thing which has great potential for immediate effect is when you discontinue foods and additives which are irritating your system. The obvious place to start here is to do your best to stop eating prepared foods which contain toxic glutamates (MSG and MSG like substances, listed later in the book) and other harmful additives.

Also there are other guidelines here that have a direct connection to immune system health. By eating freshly prepared whole foods instead of processed and modified foods, you will be intaking immune boosting anti-oxidants and discontinuing the intake of immune robbing oxidized substances. Remember that the second nature's container is broken, oxidation begins. Thus whole grains are preferable to flour products (breads, cereals, etc.), fresh fruit instead of juice, and so on. And again, the fresh low starch "Bielers" vegetables are very valuable to immune system health because of their high concentration of antioxidants and easily absorbed alkalinizing nutrients.

Finally there are a number of guidelines in this book that promote immune system health in less obvious ways. By following these you may not notice immediate improvement, but over time they can contribute significantly. An example of this might be proper food combining for efficient digestion. Besides eventually eliminating any digestion discomfort (gas, bloating, etc.), following these guidelines speeds the passage of nutrients into your bloodstream (thus reducing fatigue and stress) and frees up energy that can be better used to increase immune system health.

Recommended Reading:

Food is Your Best Medicine by Dr. Henry Bieler MD

Dr. Bieler's Natural Way to Sexual Health by Dr. Henry Bieler MD

● Diet/Low Fat Products Can Cause Problems

Snack Foods Can = Poor Health

Note: Even if you are not overweight, this section still offers a lot of important information on how your body chemistry is negatively effected by many common foods.

With so many "Low Fat" snacks and foods available in the grocery stores, many people who are trying to manage their weight naturally are attracted to these items. This is because we have been led to believe that decreasing fat intake alone will lead to weight loss and good health. Unfortunately this has not proven to be true, as people continue to carry too much weight despite consuming ever greater quantities of low fat/diet foods.

While decreasing overall fat intake is a healthy approach, there are many other aspects of body chemistry that must be addressed in order to achieve lasting success. If you simply are replacing your favorite snack foods with low fat versions, then you can cause a weight gain even if your fat and calorie intake is lower than before.

To understand why this happens you need to realize how your body is designed to work. Over thousands of years our bodies have evolved to handle sugars as they are found in their natural whole forms, namely fruits, vegetables and whole grains (not flour products). Known as complex carbohydrates, these naturally sustaining foods are absorbed gradually into the blood stream with the help of a myriad of additional nutrients that are also present in the whole foods.

Simple sugars such as table sugar (sucrose), refined fructose, barley malt, maple syrup, honey, fruit juices, fruit sweeteners and refined simple carbohydrates (flour products, especially white flour, such as breads, cereals, pasta, noodles, cakes, cookies, rice cakes, etc.) rapidly raise blood sugar when ingested. When a rapid rise in blood sugar occurs the pancreas is triggered to release a hormone called insulin. The insulin in turn moves glucose (blood sugar) out of the blood stream and into the cells, thereby regulating the circulating blood sugar.

But because this response is not instantaneous, the pancreas continues to produce insulin even as the blood sugar is dropping from the initial simple sugar/insulin reaction. The unfortunate result of all this is low blood sugar which tends to manifest as fatigue, foggy headed feeling, difficulty thinking, slow reaction and even dizziness among others.

Regrettably the reaction to the intake of the simple sugars does not stop there. In response to the drop in blood sugar, the adrenal glands begin to pump out greater quantities of the hormones adrenaline and cortisol. When your body does this it is using up precious stored energy. If this situation continues over a long period of time, the adrenals begin to wear down and conditions such as feeling chronically fatigued, anxiety and depression are the result. Also when insulin and cortisol levels are high, cholesterol increases and the kidneys retain water and salt which in turn causes the blood pressure to rise.

As with the simple sugars, the simple carbohydrates (flour) produce the same results only at a slightly slower rate (considering that most snack foods are mostly a combination of flour, sugar and salt, you can see that this is a recipe for disaster. <u>I would like to point out here that even if you do not have a weight problem, eating too much simple sugars and carbohydrates can still adversely effect your immune system.</u> This is especially so if you have immune related conditions such as allergies, asthma, chronic fatigue, fibromyalgia, lupus and other autoimmune processes including rheumatoid arthritis, irritable bowel syndrome or cancer. Now here comes the part where the weight gain happens. Once your cells are saturated with all the glucose they can handle, the overflow is transformed into fat. Sometimes overweight people will develop a condition called "insulin resistance" which occurs when insulin is unable to move glucose into the cells. Here the cells keep sending the message for more glucose so the pancreas keeps on producing more insulin, but unfortunately the cells cannot accept any more. So a vicious cycle develops where the excess glucose is converted into fat and the more "low fat" products that you eat, the fatter you get. If this cycle is not corrected, chronically high blood sugar can result in type II diabetes.

OK, so what do I do to stop this from happening you ask? Fortunately the answer is quite simple; just treat your body as it was designed. And all that means is to eat well balanced whole foods in combination with moderate, regular exercise. Doing this will balance your blood sugar and when that happens you taking a big step toward better health.

Of course this is something that you may hear all the time, but you have not quite figured out exactly how to do it or maybe it seems too hard to do. Well that is where this book comes in handy because it is full of step by step specific quidelines. This book is also <u>not</u> about deprivation, but instead is a guide to help you find pleasure and health in foods that are truly good for you. Also I believe that exercise need not be a chore, but instead is something that can be fun.

Now the importance of exercise cannot be underestimated as its benefits are HUGE. First of all it produces chemicals in your brain that contibute to wellbeing, promotes sexual energy and helps you maintain a healthy weight. Although that sounds like enough of an enticement, here are also some specifics about how exercise promotes weight loss.

When you move your body in some form of gentle, sustained exercise for at least 15-20 minutes, glucose moves into your cells without the aid of insulin. This way your blood sugar stays balanced while your pancreas and adrenals get a rest. Also when your blood sugar is reduced during exercise, your insulin secretion is suppressed and your body uses stored glucose from the muscles and liver. This in turn results in the burning of more fat.

So with all this in mind, read on and explore all the ideas presented here that will help you balance your body and your life. I realize that what you are embarking on here may not be easy for you, so I have included a vast amount of information and ideas for you to choose from. Nothing in this book is extreme or harsh, everything here is designed to bring you gently into balance and harmony. So be kind to your self along the way and let this book guide you to healthy satisfaction.

● *Food Sensitivities*

Since this book is about helping you find what foods will work best for you, it can also be seen as a system that will help you identify the foods that cause you problems. Just as the low fat / diet food problem is one mechanism that promotes poor health, there are others which we will put under the category of "food sensitivities."

Food sensitivities are a contributing factor to many people's health problems and are often a major cause of a depressed immune system. They are present or are developed for a number of reasons and even many natural whole foods can cause a reaction in a particular person.

One way people can develop food sensitivities over time is by eating only one thing and not rotating in a variety of similar foods. Many people are sensitive to such common foods as corn and wheat for this very reason.

The other causes of food sensitivities are also mostly due to poor dietary habits and they include poor digestion, nutrient deficiencies, a limited diet of highly processed foods and very often "leaky gut syndrome" (leaky gut syndrome happens when the digestive tract is too permeable and allows toxins to enter the blood stream; this syndrome is often brought on by alcohol consumption, the use of nonsteroidal anti-inflammatory drugs like aspirin, ibuprofen and acetaminophen, and assorted viral, bacterial, parasitic and yeast infections).

The following are some symptoms that people experiencing food sensitivities might exhibit:

> *water retention, tending to gain several pounds in 1-2 days; trouble losing weight through restricting calories or exercising; losing weight while dieting but unable to get past a certain point; abnormal food cravings and binge eating; mental or physical fatigue and depression; puffiness or dark circles under the eyes; excess mucus or phlegm, chronically congested nose, runny nose or post nasal drip; poor digestion, bloating, flatulence, constipation alternating with diarrhea, nausea or abdominal pains/cramps; sore achy muscles or joints; frequent headaches; mood swings, irritability, panic attacks, hyperactivity, anxiety.*

A common reaction for the food sensitive person is water retention. When partially digested food compounds pass through a compromised intestinal lining (leaky gut) into the bloodstream and eventually to the tissues, they cause irritation and inflammation. The body then attempts to reduce this irritation by diluting the offending material with fluid (note: practically all of my food sensitive clients experience immediate relief from this uncomfortable bloat when they follow the guidelines laid out in this book).

Food sensitivities can also cause problems through a process many of us are familiar with, namely food addictions. One study has found that partially digested compounds in food allergens act like morphine-like opiat drugs. This means that eating food allergens can cause a "high" that eventually wears off, thus producing a craving for more allergens in order to get back the euphoric sensation. By repeating this pattern people can become both physiologically and psychologically addicted. If a person tries eating less of these foods it's like asking an alcoholic to have one glass of wine a day. The cravings for these types of foods can become so uncontrollable that binge eating habits may develop.

Here again a lot of sobering information has been presented to you; and I would just like to say at this point that the information in this book is directly aimed at rectifying all of the conditions that you have just read about. I have seen all of these conditions before and I have also watched people say good-bye to these difficulties by changing their life-style and eating habits. Another point I want to emphasize here is that this information is not intended to replace the care and advice of medical professionals. I strongly urge you to seek the help of the qualified practitioners with whom you feel most comfortable; the information here will work well with any other treatment that you are following, consider it as a foundation for your health.

Now there are basically two ways to determine what foods you are sensitive to. The first way is to have a blood test for food allergies. This method will give you some idea at that particular point of time as to what you might be allergic to. The downside of this approach is that your body's needs change hourly, daily and seasonally. So if you choose to do this, remember that it is only a "snap shot" but it will give you some guidelines.

The second way, and the one that ultimately works because it teaches body awareness, is to keep a body feedback journal (an example is provided on p. 34). Like a diary, you simply keep track of what you eat, when you eat it and how you feel. Another advantage this system has over the first, is that you can recognize and determine delayed reactions to foods; as much of the time a reaction may take as many as three days to surface. Also you can go back in the journal and see larger, seasonal patterns. And finally your doctor or other healthcare professional will find this information very useful.

A word about "gluten free"

Many people are sensitive to a particular gluten such as wheat or grains close to wheat AND corn or soy itself. However many people may tolerate oats well even though oats are technically a gluten containing grain. So instead of avoiding all glutens, it may be a good idea to use the "Body Feedback Journal" to determine exactly which forms of gluten you react to. It is always best to try to eat the widest variety of foods possible in order to get the widest variety of nutrients.

● *What to Eat & What Not to Eat*

The Basics

The following basics are the bare bones on which you can build your own personalized "optimal" food plan. Everyone is different, and this book will help you discover what works best for you.

- **Increase in your diet lightly cooked (steamed) vegetables**

- **Eat as much <u>low starch vegetables</u> as you like.**

    The following is a partial list:

    Asparagus, Artichoke, Bok Choy, Broccoli, Brussel Sprouts, Cabbage: Napa, Red, Savoy, Cauliflower, Celery, Cilantro, Collards, Cucumber, Dandelion Greens, Endive, Eggplant, Green Beans, Kale, Leeks, Okra, Parsley, Scallions, Snow Peas, Spinach, Squash-Summer, Squash-Yellow, Squash-Zucchini, Swiss Chard, Turnip Greens.

    *Summer Squash and Zucchini are highly recommended.

- **Can have 2-4 palm size portions of <u>vegetable starch</u> or whole grain a day,**

    depending on your size, health and activity levels. <u>Do not combine with red meat</u>.

    The following is a partial list:

<u>Vegetable Starch</u>

Carrot, Beets, Corn, Legumes, Potato, Sweet Potato, Yam, Winter Squash: Acorn, Butternut, Hubbard, Spaghetti

<u>Whole Grains</u>

Rice, Spelt, Amaranth, Barley, Buckwheat, Kamut, Millet, Oatbran, Oatmeal, Quinoa, Rye, Wheat

- **Include 1-2 palm size portions of <u>protein</u> a day.** Choose from the following:

    Beef, Lamb, Chicken, Turkey, Fish (no shellfish), Buffalo, Venison (free range, ethically raised, not hormone of additive fed, is best) *Red meat is best eaten rare.

- **Can have 1-4 free range fertile eggs weekly;** treat as <u>protein</u>, <u>do not combine with meat or dairy with the exception of butter</u>.

- **Can have 1-2 servings of <u>fruit</u> daily**; cooked is better than raw for some people with sensitive digestive systems (cooked foods are easier to digest, but if you do well with some raw fruit, great!; especially during the summer when it is in season).

- **Include 1-2 Tablespoons of oil a day.** Choose from the following:

    Olive (extra virgin) ,Canola, Grapeseed, Safflower, Sunflower or Apricot Kernel (cold pressed oils are best). Also *Hazelnut, Walnut and Flax* oils are good but must be fresh and refrigerated, and remember that these oils cannot be heated.

- **Eat small regular meals. 3 meals with 1- 2 snacks is a plan that works well for many people.** The larger meals should be earlier in the day and it is best to avoid overloading at night or eating 2 hours before bed.

- **Decrease simple sugars (includes alcohol), simple carbohydrates (flour) and salt; eliminate artificial sweeteners, preservatives and chemicals.**

- **Drink enough pure (non tap) water to stay hydrated. Optimal amounts will vary from person to person.**

- **Eat a wide variety in all food groups to ensure receiving a full spectrum of nutrients.**

- **Bieler's Soup is highly recommended.** The following is the recipe:

    Ingredients:

    4-6 Zucchini sliced (medium size)

    1 lb Fresh or Frozen Green Beans

    1 Handful of Parsley Tops

    2-4 Stalks of Celery sliced <u>with strings removed</u> (Optional)

Fill a large pot with 1/3 water and add all ingredients. Cover and cook in rapidly boiling water for 15-18 minutes or until the vegetables are fork tender. Then place all ingredients in blender and <u>puree in batches until smooth</u>. Season with any of your favorite herbs, i.e., paprika, oregano, garlic, lemon or basil. Serve hot or cold. DO NOT ADD SALT.

The Specifics

Food Awareness

It is important to relax for a few minutes both before and after eating. Eating while upset, in a hurry, or while doing something else splits your attention and does not allow you to focus on the experience of enjoying your meals. Eating while stressed, or in a hurry also hinders efficient digestion of your food. Generally it is better to skip a meal rather than 'multi task' while eating

Since digestion begins in the mouth, chew your food thoroughly. Remember to slow down and stop eating before you are completely full. It takes time for the stomach to signal your brain that you've had enough. Quantity changes quality — even too much healthy food can be unhealthy.

It is best to allow at least two hours between your last meal and bedtime, so that your stomach is not full when you go to sleep.
One of the most important points in enjoying food is to release any judgement about foods. Attaching negative thoughts such as guilt over food choices, or adopting a set of rigid rules about eating places unnecessary stress on the entire system by trying to live up to unrealistic goals.

It is important to realize that the idea of "good" and "bad" foods is best viewed as a relative rather than absolute concept. Each of us is biochemically unique with needs that vary in response to our life-style, the seasons, and our environment. So what may be found to be "good" today, may be "bad" next week.

Rather than labeling foods "good" or "bad" on a solely intellectual basis, it may be more productive to release any preconceived judgements and allow your body to guide you towards what is appropriate for you now. A "Body Feedback Journal" is one way to discern what your individual needs are. A sample journal page is given on page 34.

Food Quality

Always choose foods with the least amount of processing and additives. Avoid all foods that are prepared with chemicals and preservatives. Reading labels cannot be overstressed as your best strategy for health supportive eating.

Almost every food that is processed has lost vitamins and minerals and most have salts, fats and sweeteners added to them, further insulting the body.

Buy organic grains, fruits, legumes, and vegetables whenever possible. Raw dairy products, fertile, free-range eggs, and ethically raised, chemical free meats and poultry are your best choices in the animal product category.

Ethically raised, chemical free meats and poultry are in many ways healthier than "factory farmed" animals. Factory farmed animals lead a very stressful existence and accumulate poisons associated with that stress. Because their immune systems are so hampered from stress, they need large amounts of antibiotics and chemicals in their feed which are ultimately passed on to the human consumer. In contrast, ethically raised animals are usually raised in the U.S., and therefore do not contribute to the deforestation of central and South America for grazing land.

Your first and best choice in all food categories is fresh. If for some reason that is not available, frozen organic and standard frozen are the next best option, but always read the labels and check for additives. In a pinch, canned no salt food is better than nothing at all, but again, read the labels carefully.

Because our air, soil and ground water is not as pure as it was as little as 30 years ago, it is a prudent idea to eat a wide variety of foods in order to avoid the chemical residues that a specific food would uptake. Even organically grown produce can be affected by the chemicals used previously in the soil, pesticide drift from neighboring farms, and groundwater seepage and rainfall.

Water

Drink enough pure water to stay hydrated. Optimal amounts vary with the individual, seasons and activity levels. However avoid drinking with meals. Large amounts of liquids, of any variety, consumed in conjunction with your meals can hinder digestion and contribute to an uncomfortable bloated feeling.

Eat Seasonally and Locally

Mother nature, in her infinite wisdom, has provided the appropriate foods at the appropriate time of year to keep your body in tune with the seasons and your environment. If the food is in season, grows locally or is from a similar climate zone, it is probably a health-enhancing choice.

Cooking Consciously

The manner in which you prepare your foods and the utensils you cook in all have an affect on the end product. Your preparation time can be used as a break to wind down before eating, so relax and enjoy what you are doing.

To prevent potentially toxic minerals from leaching into your foods, cook in pyrex, corning ware, stainless steel, or lead free earthenware.

Conscious use of cooking techniques can also alter the energetic quality of a food which directly affects the way you feel. Generally speaking, cooking at high temperatures for long periods of time (i.e. baking, roasting, barbecuing) will make foods relatively more energizing and more dry, while stewing over low-heat for a long period of time makes foods more moist and easily digestible. Steaming or parboiling creates a lighter quality and makes foods easier to digest than large amounts of raw foods.

Vegetables

Fresh vegetables should be eaten as the predominant food group in all diets. Vegetables are a storehouse of many important vitamins and minerals as well as a great source of fiber. This category can be thought of as the balancers in the nutrition equation.

It is also very important to eat a wide variety of fresh vegetables. Fortunately there are so many varieties available that one could never become bored. Buy "organically grown" whenever possible or at least wash thoroughly.

The following is partial list:

Green and Low Starch Vegetables

Alfalfa Sprouts, Other Sprouts, Asparagus, Artichoke, Avocado (in moderation as it is very high in fat), Beet Greens, Bell Peppers, Bok Choy, Broccoli, Brussel Sprouts, Cabbage: Napa, Red, Savoy.

Cauliflower, Celery, Cilantro , Collards, Cucumber, Dandelion Greens, Endive, Eggplant, Garlic , Green Beans,

Kale Jerusalem Artichokes, Leeks, Mung Bean Sprouts, Mushrooms, Mustard Greens, Radish, Okra, Onions, Parsley, Scallions,Snow Peas

Spinach , Squash-Summer, Squash-Yellow,Squash-Zucchini, Swiss Chard, Tomato, Turnip Greens, Watercress, Lettuce: Bibb, Butter, Iceberg, Red Leaf, Romaine

Vegetable Starch

Beet, Legumes, Carrots, Corn, Garbanzo Beans, Jicama, Lentils, Lima Beans, Parsnip, Peas, Potato , Sweet Potato, Turnip, Yam,

Winter Squash: Acorn, Butternut, Hubbard,Spaghetti

Proteins

The average adult needs far less protein than we are accustomed to consuming. Use all protein sources as side dishes, relying on fresh vegetables and whole grains as the center of your meals. One to two palm sized portions of protein per day (adjusted to individual needs) with at least twice the amount of fresh low starch vegetables and appropriate amounts of grain / starchy vegetables is a health supportive balance.

If you choose to include animal proteins in your diet, buy the leanest cut and remove all visible skin and fat. The fatty portions contain the highest residues of any chemicals, hormones and antibiotics used on the animal as well as being high in saturated fats.

Fish and seafood must be chosen carefully. Be sure to ask where the fish was caught and if they were dipped in antibiotics or preservatives upon catch. When buying canned tuna, be sure to buy "dolphin safe." Because our oceans and lakes are so polluted, only occasional use of bottom feeders, the category of scavenging fish or shellfish is best. Also farm raised fish produces another set of issues because of the manner in which they are raised. Do your research because some farm raised sources are better than others.

The following is a partial list:

Beef, Beef Liver (organically rasied only), Beef Veal, Buffalo, Chicken , Duck, Eggs, Fish, Goose, Lamb, Nuts, Seeds, Tofu, Turkey, Venison. *Red meat is best eaten rare

Grains and Flour Products

Eat a wide variety of grains and make your first choice whole and unprocessed grain. Flour products, even if they are made from whole grains, should be used as an adjunct. Flour products such as crackers, pastas, and breads usually have salt, fats and many forms of sweeteners added to them, so read labels carefully. Also when grains are milled, vitamins and minerals are lost and natural oils can more easily oxidize. Furthermore, the longer the flour sits before baking, and the longer the finished product sits on the shelf before consumption, the more vitamin loss and oxidation takes place. Grain intake needs to be adjusted to your individual activity level. If you lead a physically active life-style, increase grain portions accordingly.

The following is a partial list:

Grains

Amaranth, Barley, Buckwheat, Corn, Kamut, Millet, Oatbran, Oatmeal, Quinoa, Rice, Rye, Spelt, Wheat

Breads

Kamut, Spelt, Rye, Millet, Sour Dough, Wheat, Rice Bread, Rice Cakes, Pastas (yeast free breads are best)

Legumes

Legumes (beans, peas, lentils), properly prepared, are an optional protein source, especially for people with high physical activity levels. If there is a tendency towards digestive problems (i.e. recurrent bloating, indigestion after meals) you may want to use this food group with discretion. Do not combine legumes with animal protein or dairy. Dr. Bieler recommended certain legumes to normalize the sex glands (See p. 213 in *Natural Way To Sexual Health* for more information).

Legumes can be made more easily digestible if soaked in water overnight and can be cooked in fresh water slowly over low heat for 3-4 hours. Kombu (a type of seaweed popular in Japan) may be added at the beginning of cooking to add flavor and minerals, and make them even more digestible.

As with any protein, be sure to have at least twice the amount of low starch vegetables per serving of protein. Legume amounts may be increased to slightly more than a palm sized portion with an equal amount (or slightly more) of a whole grain and vegetable starch. These proportions again would vary according to individual activity levels.

Fruits

It is always best to eat organic, whole, fresh fruit. Choose what is in season and native to your climate zone. Be sure to wash thoroughly all fruits, especially non-organic. Even though fresh, whole fruit contains a natural form of sugar, this food group should be thought of as a snack or a dessert, not the center of your diet. Dried fruits are a very concentrated form of fruit sugar, so moderation is necessary. Also melons deserve some explanation as they are quite a complex food. If you are experiencing less than optimal health they are best avoided and remember to eat them in season. If you drink fruit juice always dilute 50/50 with water.

The following is a partial list:

Apple, Apricot, Banana, Blackberry, Blueberry, Boysenberry, Cherimoya, Cherry, Cranberry, Dried Fruit, Elderberry , Fig, Gooseberry

Grapefruit, Grapes, Guava, Kiwi, Kumquat, Lemon, Lime, Loganberry, Mango, Nectarine, Orange, Papaya, Peach, Pear

Persimmon, Pineapple, Plum, Pomegranate, Raspberry, Strawberry, Tangerine

Dairy Products*

When using dairy products your first choice should be raw, low-fat in some cases, and low sodium as applicable. When selecting cheeses make sure they are rennetless (for easier digestion) and free from dyes or chemicals. Many adults do not handle dairy products (with the exception of butter) well, so use your discretion. However some people can handle goats milk products more easily than cows milk derivations.

Note that eggs are not considered a dairy product.

The following is a partial list:

*Cheese, *Cottage Cheese, *Cream, *Cream Cheese, Kefir, Milk, Yogurt*

* indicates not for daily use

Food Combining Awareness for Healthy Digestion

If you are experiencing less than radiant health we have found that keeping the combinations of foods simple gives the body a chance to restore balance more easily. For some this may mean following these guidelines most of the time and for others maybe only one or two points will be necessary to maintain well-being. Much depends on your physical activity, lifestyle, reactions to life situations, age and season of the year as to what will work for you.

Please allow yourself to be flexible with your food choices as things change in your life, adapting the ideas in this book to suit your circumstances. Let your body be your guide in selecting what supports your individual needs at the time by utilizing the body feedback journal in this book. Your body will always tell you what can be handled.

• It is best to combine only one type of protein at a time per meal, ie. no eggs and steak (or breakfast meat), no cheese and meat, no eggs and cheese, no steak and shrimp, etc.

• When eating beef, lamb, liver, or veal, most people do well to avoid combining them with grains (rice, etc.), flour products (bread, chips, etc.) or starches (potatoes, etc.). This means avoiding hamburgers and french fries, lamb and potatoes, and beef and pasta. Beef, lamb, liver, veal and eggs also do not combine well with dairy products; this includes butter. When you eat red meat combine it only with low starch vegetables and nothing else (adding a small amount of oil to flavor is OK). This is a flexible point as some people when healthy do fine combining red meat with grains / flour products / vegetable starch.

- Wait at approximately 1 1/2 hours between meals and snacks.

- Wait at least 1 1/2 hours between eating vegetables and fruits. The only exceptions to this are lemons, limes and apples.

- Eat bananas alone and melons by themselves, as they are complex foods and may overload the system when combined with other foods.

- When eating chicken, turkey, fish or eggs, they combine well with grains, flour products, starchy vegetables and low starch vegetables for most people.

- Small amounts of fruit with grains or flour products and fruit with diary will also combine fairly well.

- Protein can also combine with fruit.

Fats

All fats should be used sparingly, as they are a highly concentrated food and tend to congest the system if done to excess. Mayonnaise, butter (which is preferable to margarine), oils, coconut, avocado, nuts, nut and seed butters, and seeds all fall into this category. Read all labels carefully and be on the alert for hidden fats in packaged foods (i.e. breads, crackers, cookies, granola, and prepackaged cereals).

For adults in good health, 1 - 2 Tbls of added fat can be included daily if you eat animal protein, and 3 - 4 Tbls of added fat daily it you are vegetarian.

In the oil category, always buy cold-pressed oils and extra-virgin olive oil. Date all your oils, refrigerate, and discard them after 3 months,. Oils oxidize and become rancid when exposed to heat and/or light. When selecting a cooking oil, mono-unsaturated or high oleic oils are more molecularly stable than other oils at higher temperatures. Vary your intake of polyunsaturated oils as all provide a different balance of fatty acids to the body.

The following is a partial list:

> *Butter, Mayonnaise, Nut Butters, Oils: extra virgin Olive ,Canola, Grape Seed, Safflower, Sunflower, Apricot Kernel, Hazelnut, Walnut, Flax, Pumpkin Seed* (cold pressed oils are best).

Avoid Hydrogenated Fats and Oils like Shortenings and Margarine

Trans Fatty Acids are formed when fats and oils are hydrogenated. During this process hydrogen molecules are added to polyunsaturated or monounsaturated oils, which then creates semisolid shortenings or margarines. The bad news here is that this modification makes the fat very difficult to digest. Furthermore many studies have now proven that these trans fatty acids unbalance the cholesterol in the blood which in turn leads to a variety of problems.

Now we have all heard a lot about cholesterol, but unfortunately most of the information provided is over simplified and not complete. Consequently perceptions such as, "cholesterol is this awful, gummy stuff clogs up arteries which leads to heart attacks," or "every time you eat food that contains cholesterol your cholesterol levels rise," are only half truths. So let's take a look here at the whole truth so we can understand how things really work.

What is Cholesterol?

Cholesterol is the mother of all hormones. Specifically it is a fat-soluble steroid that is the basis for all steroid hormones. Cholesterol is also a very important component of the brain, as it is part of the myelin sheath that protects nerves and nerve impulse propagation. Therefore it makes sense that if your cholesterol levels are too low, both your hormone balance and brain function suffer. So you can see that cholesterol is not bad in itself and is in fact both important and necessary to support healhy body functions.

Eating food with cholesterol in it does not in itself cause chronically high cholesterol levels. In humans, a large portion of our cholesterol is synthesized in the liver from sugars and dietary fats. Diets with a high intake of simple sugars will cause high cholesterol as well as eating cholesterol laden food. Also it is important to realize that stress elevates cholesterol tremendously.

Problems begin when the relationship between the different types of cholesterol becomes unbalanced. The cholesterol in your bloodstream is attached to one of several different molecules. Two of these molecules are high density lipoproteins (HDL) and low density lipoproteins (LDL). Now the mere presence of HDL and LDL is fine, but bad things start to happen when HDL levels get too low or LDL levels get too high. This is because HDL protects the more fragile LDL from being oxidized. If the LDL oxidizes, then arterial plaque that clogs arteries is usually the result.

So what can you do to keep this from happening? Simple, eat more low starch vegetables which are full of antioxidants and avoid hydrogenated oils which are full of trans fatty acids (rancid artery cloggers). Also intake a small amount of fats and oils that are that are natural and complex. This means eating lean free range meats, poultry and fish, and cold pressed oils like olive, coconut, high oleic sunflower, high oleic safflower, almond, apricot kernel, etc. (avoid peanut).

Salt

Fresh vegetables, proteins, grain and fruits provide all the natural sodium necessary for balance within the body. All forms of salt (i.e., sea salt, miso, tamari, and soy sauce) should be used with a very light hand and cooked into foods, not added at the table. It is best to use these condiments for special occasions, not daily use.

There are a number of reasons why salt in its processed inorganic crystalline form should be mostly avoided. Basically what excess salt does is cause the deterioration of your vital organs, especially the liver and the kidneys. It also interferes with the elimination of certain waste products of the metabolism.

So why do we eat it and why are so many people hooked on it? Quite simply the answer is that it is a stimulant. In the same way that people use simple sugars, simple carbohydrates (flour) and caffeine, people use salt to give them a temporary energy boost because their nutrient poor, unbalanced eating habits are not giving them what they need. Unfortunately this short term stimulant strategy in the long run leads to all the ailments that we see in young and old alike today.

Fortunately, by reading and understanding this, you can act to change your habits and most likely avoid these problems. Here is a sobering figure that the U.S government and most scientists believe is true, that 75% of the disease in the U.S. is preventable and can be avoided through life-style/habit change.

So here is all you have to remember, your body needs organic sodium that is naturally found in vegetables (zucchini and other green low starch vegetables mostly), not processed sodium chloride in its crystalline forms of table salt. Celtic salt, which contains many beneficial minerals, may be an exception for some people if it is used occasionally and in very small amounts (1-2 pinches a day).

Caffeine

Caffeine should be greatly reduced or eliminated from most diets. Not only does it deplete the body of many important "B" group vitamins, but it also may increase an individual's susceptibility to coronary heart disease, if so predisposed. Caffeine also hyper-stimulates the adrenal glands which over time can seriously deplete them. Coffee, black tea, diet sodas and most chocolates fall into this category. Think of using some of the many varieties of herbal teas available as a substitute.

Concentrated Sugars

Refined sugars such as white sugar, molasses, corn syrup, and fructose, as well as all artificial sweeteners should be avoided. These have no nutritional value, providing only "empty" calories. Artificial sweeteners have also been implicated in many health problems.

Honey, agave, maple sugar, date sugar, barley-malt, rice-syrup, rice bran syrup, and fruit juice concentrates are very concentrated forms of naturally occurring sugars, so should be used in moderation.

For general use, in order of preference, try stevia, fruit juice concentrates, agave, rice syrup, rice bran syrup or powder, barley malt, maple sugar, date sugar, and finally, honey.

It is nearly impossible to kick the sugar habit while constantly tasting a substitute, even if it is a naturally formed one. For help with strong sweet cravings, try fresh, ripe seasonal fruit. Fruit cooked with a variety of spices is also nice for a change of pace, especially in the cooler months of the year.

The wonderful exceptionally sweet tasting root called *Stevia* can help with sweet cravings and does not raise blood sugar levels. It does not always do well in baking recipes but is quite good sprinkled on things or in drinks. It is highly concentrated so very little is needed for effect. It is also now conveniently available in a white powdered form in individual packets (just like artificial sweetener packets).

Alcohol

Like refined sugar, this substance also provides calories without nutritional benefits. Alcohol is even more rapidly converted in the body than refined sugar, reeking havoc with blood sugar levels. The deleterious effects of alcohol on various organs in the body as well as the consciousness are very well documented.

Harmful Additives to Avoid

Glutamates

Glutamates are commonly found in the vast majority of prepared foods, even health food brands. Toxicologists point out that glutamates are neuro-toxins and are harmful to everyone. The following is a partial list of many types of glutamates:

> *MSG, Accent, autolyzed yeast, ajinomoto, aspartame (acts like MSG), barley malt, malt extract, broth, bouillon, Chinese seasoning, carrageenan, calcium caseinate, disodium guanylate, disodium inosinate, dough conditioners, flavorings, natural flavorings (not all), flavors (i.e. turkey flavor), flutacyl, glutavene, gourmet powder, gelatin, hydrolyzed protein, hydrolyzed plant protein, hydrolyzed vegetable protein, hydrolyzed milk protein, kombu extract, L-Cysteine, monosodium glutamate, mono potassium glutamate, Mei-Jing, maltextrin, protein hydrolysate, RL-50, spices???, soy protein isolate, soy protein concentrate, soy sauce, Subu, sodium caseinate, smoke flavor, textured protein, vegetable broth, vegetable powder, vetsin, whipping agents, Wei-Jing, whey protein concentrate, protein isolate, yeast extract, zest.* * Note: Artificial sweeteners such as aspartame, NutraSweet, Sweet and Low are very harmful. It is better to eat sugar than to put these toxins into your system.

Eating Out

Caution and questions are the keys to health supportive dining. Always ask if MSG is used, or if sugar and salt are added. Find out how the food is prepared and where it comes from. If the waitress of waiter is not sure, have them ask the chef. Also ask for sauces and dressings on the side. Most restaurants will accommodate you, especially if you have food sensitivities.

Where to Shop

Your local health food store is by far the best place to shop. There are now health food stores in just about every city and most larger towns. However, you may be disappointed to find that some "health food" stores are actually little more than vitamin stores.

Your health food store should carry foods that are not highly processed, organically grown produce and grains, and ethically raised, chemical free meats and poultry. Ethically raised means that the animals were not "factory farmed," or cruelly treated, and were fed a rich and healthy natural diet, instead of one full of junk, hormones and antibiotics. Chickens should be cage-free and their eggs should be fertile. It is beyond the scope of this book to delve deeply into the ethical, moral, and environmental issues of food. There are several excellent books available at your local health food store on these topics.

One common fallacy about health food stores is that the food is often more expensive. Because a health supportive diet should include more fresh foods than processed foods, it costs less than the typical diet.

If you are not fortunate enough to live close to a health food store you can also approach your local supermarket managers and ask them to carry the foods you would like to buy. Fortunately many major chains now have health food sections and carry organic produce. Of course this is because customers such as yourself have asked for this

Beware of health claims made on products from non health food stores. Claims such as "90% Fat Free," "No Preservatives," "No added sugar," "30% less calories," "Diet," "Sugar Free," etc., may mean very little for your health. A preservative free bread, for example, may have dough conditioners, sugar and added fat. A product with 30% less calories probably had 80% too many to begin with, and to cover up the lost flavor, may use other undesirable additives. Diet and Sugar Free products may have artificial sweeteners. Be a conscientious label reader. Otherwise, you'll never know what you're getting.

Some of the brands listed next may not be available at your local health food store. These are brands that are available in the Los Angeles area, that we have found to be consistently good quality, without unnecessary additives. Other brands may be equally good. Just be sure to check the ingredients on the label. Remember they are listed in decreasing order of amount, so the biggest ingredient is listed first.

Condiments, Seasonings and Spices

While it is ok to enjoy condiments, seasonings and spices occasionally, it is best to stick with a squeeze of lemon or lime, dried and fresh herbs and in some cases a small amount of vinegar for daily use when restoring health. Here is a list of "*the extras*" for non-regular use according to individual need:

    Amasake
    Black or White Pepper
    Cayenne Pepper
    Mirin
    Worchestshire Sauce
    Mustard / Wasabi
    Miso
    Garlic
    Onions

Simple Substitutions: Instead of . . .

* indicates not for daily use

Diet Sodas:

Perrier or mineral water with 1/2 glass of apple juice, white or purple grape juice, cranberry concentrate, or any of your favorite juices.

Pasta*:

Soba (100% buckwheat), kamut, spelt, and rice pastas are a nice alternative to wheat based pastas (health food stores carry them in the oriental section). Rice noodles (available in health food stores), eggless noodles, Jerusalem artichoke noodles, eggless lasagna, fresh egg white based pasta.

Sweeteners:

Fruit juice concentrates (Hain, Mystic Lakes), Unsweetened frozen fruit juices (use full strength), pureed cooked or fresh, unsweetened frozen fruits. Amasake* (a cultured rice product), barley or rice syrup* (Yinnies, Mitoku, Sweet Cloud, Eden), Stevia (both liquid and powder).

Butter/Jams:

Unsweetened applesauce with or without cinnamon, homemade fruit purees or compotes, unsweetened or fruit juice sweetened preserves, (L.A., Sorrell Ridge, Westbrae, Poiret), unsweetened apple butter (L.A., Westbrae, Eden).

Non Yeasted Breads:

Corn tortillas, rice cakes (Lundbergs [the crunchiest], Arden, Hain, Chicosan, Pritikin), Ponce breads, Lotus breads, Rudolphs all rye bread, Essene sprouted, unbaked at high heat breads (Essene, Garden of Eatin, Lifestream, Manna), mochi (pounded sweet rice cake). Mystic Lakes rice bread, Foods for Life rice bread. Pacific Bakeries or French Meadows kamut or spelt bagels and breads.

Sour Cream:

Lowfat yogurt mixed with herbs and spices.

Cheeses*:

Rennetless, raw, low-fat, low or no sodium.

Milk on Cereals:

Soy milk. rice milk, oat milk, amasake, fruit juices (try mixing rice and oat for richer taste). unsweetened coconut milk.

Salad Dressing:

Try low oil or unsweetened health food brands.

Catsup/Tomato Sauce:

Try any of the health food store brands (Fruit juice sweetened, no salt is best).

Coffee Substitutes:

Emer-Gen C decafinated coffee with vitamins by Alacer, Cafe Roma, Caffix, grain based teas, Mugicha (roasted barley tea - health food store, oriental section), Dacopa, Creamy Carob herbal teas, Yogi teas.

Chocolate Substitutes*:

Unsweetened carob powder, or unsweetened carob chips, candy bars, patties (rice, almond, or raisin crisps).

Mustard*:

Low or no sodium mustard (health food stores).

Cooking Wine*:

Mirin (a Japanese liquid seasoning found in health food stores — Eden, Mitoku brands).

Ice Cream/Sherbets*:

Rice Dream, Nouvelle Sorbet, Cafe Glace, Garden of Eatin Glace.

Waffles*:

Van's oat bran with raisins, seven-grain. Rice flour waffles, wheat-free waffle mixes.

Cookies*:

Mrs. Denesons, Pamelas and Barbaras brands all have wheat free and fruit juice sweetened recipes. Also try bread or toast with a little butter and fruit conserve or stevia powder and cinnamon.

Crackers:

Kalvi Crispbread, Wasa Rye, Wasa Lite Rye, Finn Crisps (the Wasa brand also has yeast free).

● *Other Toxins To Avoid*

If You Smoke

Of course we all know that smoking is not good for anyone, but we also know that nicotine is one of the hardest addictions to overcome. Fortunately there are a number of effective methods that can help such as acupuncture, Jin Shin Jyutsu and hypnosis. So with that in mind I would like to present some "positive" motivational information that will help you realize the specific benefits of quitting. It is never too late!

<u>Quitting smoking is the single greatest thing you can do to improve your health.</u>

When smokers quit, within <u>20 minutes of smoking that last cigarette</u>, the body begins a series of changes that continue for years:

<u>20 minutes</u> - blood pressure drops to normal, body temperature of hands and feet increases to normal, pulse rate drops to normal

<u>8 hours</u> - carbon monoxide level in blood drops to normal, oxygen level in blood increase to normal

<u>24 hours</u> - chance of heart attack decreases

<u>48 hours</u> - nerve endings start regrowing, the ability to smell and taste is enhanced

<u>2 weeks to 3 months</u> - circulation improves, walking becomes easier, lung function increases up to 30 %

<u>1 to 9 months</u> - coughing, sinus congestion, fatigue, shortness of breath decreases, cilia regrow in lungs, increasing the ability to handle mucus, clean the lungs and reduce infection

<u>1 year</u> - excess risk of heart disease is half that of a smoker

<u>5 years</u> - lung cancer death rate for average smoker (1 pack a day) decreases by half, stroke risk is reduced to that of a nonsmoker 5-15 years after quitting, risk of cancer of the mouth, throat, esophagus is half that of a smoker

<u>10 years</u> - lung cancer death rate similar to that of a nonsmoker, precancerous cells are replaced, risk of cancer of the mouth, throat, esophagus, bladder, kidney and pancreas decreases

<u>15 years</u> - risk of coronary heart disease is that of a nonsmoker

Some Basic Tools for Quitting

Stay in the moment. When a life situation triggers you acknowledge that trigger and do some Jin Shin Jyutso or take a walk to reconnect to your body.

Take a breather, literally, a few conscious breaths while doing self help Jin shin Jyutsu can head off most cravings. Relaxation exercise like yoga and Qigong help relieve urges to smoke; remember that urges to smoke are temporary, stay in the moment!

Exercise, moderate aerobic exercise like walking, bicycling and swimming will help relieve tension and your urge to smoke

Quitting Tips

Enjoy nibbling on items like carrots, celery or apples, or suck on cinnamon sticks

Stretch out your meals, pause between bites

After dinner, instead of a cigarette, treat yourself to a mint or a cup of herb tea

Skin Exposure

Your skin is the largest organ in your body and is also part of your "intake" system. This means that whatever you come into physical contact with can enter you system thorough your skin because skin is permeable. So it makes sense to be as careful here as you are with what goes into your mouth.

Of course we all know that it is wise to limit contact with obviously harmful chemicals such as solvents and strong cleaners, etc., but unfortunately there are some other toxic chemicals that are not as obvious hiding in <u>cosmetics, shampoos and skin lotions</u>. The following is a partial list with short descriptions:

<u>Isopropyl Alcohol (SD40)</u> - A petroleum derivative, drying and irritating solvent; can cause headaches, dizziness, depression, nausea and worse; fatal ingested dose is 1 oz. or less; alternative is BGSE.

<u>DEA (diethonelamine), MEA (monoethanolamine, TEA (triethnolamine)</u> - Hormone disrupting
chemicals that can form cancer causing nitrates and nitrosamines; these chemicals are already restricted in Europe because of known carcinogenic effects.

<u>DMDM Hydantoin & Urea (Imidazolidinyl)</u> - Preservatives that often release formaldehyde which may cause joint pain, skin reactions, sensitivities, depression, headaches, chest pains, ear infections, chronic fatigue, dizziness, and loss of sleep. Exposure may also irritate the respiratory system, trigger heart palpitations or asthma, and aggravate coughs and colds. Other possible side effects include weakening the immune system and cancer. Alternative: Lonicera Japonica

FD&C Color Pigments - Synthetic colors made from coal tar, containing heavy metal salts that deposit toxins onto the skin, causing skin sensitivity and irritation. Animal studies have shown almost all of them to be carcinogenic.

Synthetic Fragrances - Many toxic or carcinogenic; symptoms reported to the FDA include headaches, dizziness, allergic rashes, skin discoloration, violent coughing and vomiting, and skin irritation; clinical observation proves fragrances can affect the central nervous system, causing depression, hyperactivity, irritability, inability to cope, and other behavioral changes; alternatives: Aromatherapeutic, Organic Essential Oils.

Mineral Oil - Petroleum by-product that coats the skin like plastic, clogging the pores; interferes with skin's ability to eliminate toxins, promoting acne and other disorders; slows down skin function and cell development, resulting in premature aging; used in many products (baby oil is 100% mineral oil!); alternatives: Moisture Magnets (Saccharide Isomerate) from beets; Ceramides, Jojoba and other vegetable oils, etc.

Polyethylene Glycol (PEG) - Potentially carcinogenic petroleum ingredient used in cleansers to dissolve oil and grease; also used in caustic spray-on oven cleaners; one alternative: Planteren™.

Propylene Glycol (PG) and Butylene Glycol - Gaseous hydrocarbons which can weaken protein and cellular structure; commonly used to make extracts from herbs; the EPA considers PG so toxic that it requires workers to wear protective gloves, clothing and goggles and to dispose of any PG solutions by burying them in the ground; because PG penetrates the skin so quickly, the EPA warns against skin contact to prevent consequences such as brain, liver, and kidney abnormalities, but there isn't even a warning label on products such as stick deodorants, where the concentration is greater than in most industrial applications; alternatives: water extracted herbs, Essential Oils, etc.

Sodium Lauryl Sulfate (SLS) & Sodium Laureth Sulfate (SLES) - Detergents and surfactants used in car washes, garage floor cleaners and engine degreasers - and in 90% of personal-care products that foam; animals exposed to SLS experience eye damage, depression, labored breathing, diarrhea, severe skin irritation, and even death; when combined with other chemicals, SLS can be transformed into nitrosamines, a potent class of carcinogens. Your body may retain the SLS for up to five days, during which time it may enter and maintain residual levels in the heart, liver, the lungs, and the brain; alternative: Ammonium Cocoyl Isethionate.

Triclosan - A synthetic "antibacterial" ingredient which the EPA registers it as a pesticide, giving it high scores as a risk to both human health and the environment; it is classified as a chlorophenol, a class of chemicals suspected of causing cancer in humans; alternative: BGSE

Exposure to Human Made EMF

Human made Electrical Magnetic Frequencies (EMF) are all around us, especially those of us who live in dense urban areas. Science is trying to determine exactly how EMF affects humans but it is generally conceded that too much EMF is quite harmful to any living organic being. At its very worse it can promote cancer and at its least it can be a stress producing irritant (but don't think too lightly of stress as it is now recognized as one of the foremost causes of disease).

Human made EMF has many sources which include CRT's (cathode ray tubes. ie. computer monitors, TV's), microwaves, cell phones, fluorescent lights, power lines, etc. Since these are common and useful fixtures of modern life, completely eliminating them would not work for most people. Fortunately if precautions are taken, most people can minimize the negative effects of these things.

So how can you protect yourself from human made EMF? Well the simplest and most effective tool is to limit your exposure. The most obvious way to do this is to not spend a lot of time using or in the proximity of these devices. Secondly, when you do use EMF emitting appliances, keep a good distance between you and it (ie. don't stand right next to the microwave). Fortunately most EMF generated by appliances dissipates rapidly beyond 2-3 feet. So some other good strategies here are to watch TV from across the room, place your computer monitor at the far end of the desk and put your computer on the other side of the room (you can usually run about 8 ft. of cable extensions without loss of monitor clarity).

That sounds like some good advice you might say, but what if I have to work in environment with a lot of computers and other equipment? Well first of all there are some things like monitor screens that may help, but primarily I would recommend getting some nifty little personal EMF protection devices from The Energy Works (email: **energyworks@earthlink.net** website: **http://www.energy-works.net**). These handy things can be worn or placed in your environment to effectively neutralize human made EMF.

● Psychological & Emotional Factors

How To Satisfy Yourself On All Levels

This may be the most important part of the book. Whether we realize it or not, food and our eating habits have a prominent emotional psychological component. This is so for at least three reasons. First, the chemicals in foods influence moods and emotions; second, internal/hormonal imbalances which cause erratic mood swings and depression can be created by poor, nutrient deficient diets; and third, we often turn to food as a way to find pleasure and enjoyment when other areas of our lives are not working well for us. The first two aspects are what most of this book is about, namely how to keep your body chemically balanced and healthy so that it will help you feel good on all levels. For many people this does the trick, they change their eating habits and life-style and their whole life turns around. But many other people who are dealing with important life issues will need to consider how these things are connected with their eating habits, and that is what this chapter will discuss.

So what is the mechanism at work here in the food/emotion relationship? Simply stated, it can perhaps be best describe by the one word "nourishment." Explaining the concept of nourishment in its broadest sense, we can see it as the effort to satisfy and nurture all aspects of ourselves, from our soul to our body. If our soul is nourished, then all is well. How we choose to live and what we choose to eat are all then decisions that we make from a foundation of well being. However if something is not right in our inner world, then we often are inclined to make up for it in the outer world by desperately seeking to fill this void with sensual stimulation. In terms of food and eating this means choosing "comfort" snacks like chocolate, ice cream, donuts, etc. that provide a temporary emotional and energetic lift.

Unfortunately, as I explain in detail in the rest of this book, these short term stimulants lead to serious long term problems. So now that you have a basic understanding of this situation, you can see how important it is to nourish all aspects of yourself, taking care of each in its own way.

Before I go on further about emotion/eating specifics, I would like to take time here to address what I see as the root cause of unhappiness and therefore most people's difficulties. Life can be very challenging and often our responses to these challenges can be very upsetting. So how is it that some people smile and whistle through these things and others become depressed? After all there are many people with terminal diseases who are rays of light in this world. How do they do it?

Well I believe it is because they have connected with their 'True Self'. When you fulfill your inner purpose, which is connecting with your True Self, you can then bring forth this True Self into every aspect of your life. You are an expression of that Self in whatever life situation you find yourself in. Your outer purpose, what you do for money, what you do for fun, who you marry, etc., then becomes a vehicle for expressing your Soul. Through societal, cultural and familial conditioning so many of us get stuck in counterfeit responses to life situations that are not really 'us'. Once you are able to consistently and consciously connect with your True Self, all of these layers will simply fall away. There are many paths to achieve this end. Explore the many self awareness and spiritual development tools that are available to find what works for you.

I find that the ancient Oriental self awareness and self healing art of Jin Shin Jyutsu combined with the work of Eckhart Tolle and Byron Katie provides that path of connection for me and many of my clients. When you connect with your True Self, food then becomes one of the many sensual pleasures that you can enjoy as a human and not just a temporary fix that can never truly fulfill you. The following are a few ideas that may help you:

- Be kind to yourself, this process may take time and it will go easier if you focus on acceptance rather than criticism.

- Eat for enjoyment and hunger, not because you see it as the only way to 'fill' for yourself.

- Eat until satisfied, but if you want to eat more try to determine the reason why, if you can understand this you might figure out how to fulfill this need in a better way; perhaps you are tired or thirsty and need a nap or some water, maybe you want affection from another (spouse, child, animal), possibly exercise like a brisk walk will hit the spot, or maybe you need to connect with your inner self.

This Process of Change, How to Handle The Cravings

The following is the loving guidance of Eileen Poole, who was a student and patient of Dr. Henry Bieler, the author of *Food Is Your Best Medicine*. (Reprinted here with Eileen Poole's permission)

Dear Friend,

People come to see me for many reasons but generally speaking they want to feel better. As it is impossible to cover everything here, I still think that this information may answer most of your questions.

First of all, I am not happy with the word "diet." It sounds rather rigid and also has a temporary ring to it. After all, eating properly for your particular needs is simply a common sense *way of life*. Most people after they start the change of eating well will feel better, stronger, less tired and may not experience any discomforts at all. However others do experience various changes within a few days and many questions may arise.

All of us are different yet we have much in common. Most of us love to eat and are addicted to certain foods and have been in the habit of using a fair amount of salt and sugar in some form. These habits go back for years. Frequently from the time we are born, food has been used for many reasons. Certainly hunger has little to do with most of our eating patterns, but this we often have yet to learn. I remember as a small child my grandfather giving me rich doughnuts as treats daily. When I would end up in the hospital with severe ear problems, out of love and sympathy I would be rewarded with more treats; not aware that it was the excess sugar and fats in my small body that had created the trouble in the first place. Even going to the zoo, museums and church outings represented ice cream, etc. It's no wonder that I became hooked at an early age. So often we are trying to fill an emotional void and it can be a bottomless pit. I can remember many times sitting down to eat and not wanting ever to stop. The satisfaction was in the eating, not in the food itself. I was not experiencing smell, taste or even touch but just the anxiety of never getting enough. That is why many of us eat too quickly. The action of "shoveling it in" is to fill that void which of course can never be filled by eating. It will in fact only perpetuate it. Oddly enough, although this has been a lifetime habit, we only seem to become aware of it as we make our positive changes.

You may experience cravings, but if you understand the body will often crave the very food that it is cleansing from the system, it will make it easier to resist. However, if you give in don't let it throw you. Just understand what is happening and you will soon get back on track. I might add that many people have not eaten junk foods and been careful in their eating habits, yet they still do not feel as well as they would like. In these cases it simply has been not making the right choices for them, hence the expression, "one man's meat is another man's poison." I get many frantic calls from people in such despair because they have "gone off their diet." Not only do they feel uncomfortable physically but they fee quite wretched mentally too. The guilt reaction can be more negative and damaging than eating the incorrect food. So when we "go off" we should observe what is happening, have understanding, and then it is easier to get back on track. As time goes on this will happen less and less because our want and needs become one, which in turn makes life so much easier.

Many of us also have the habit of eating too quickly and too much. It is not likely that we will change overnight, but I assure you change *will* occur. No doubt in the beginning you will do as I did in those early days and eat large amounts of the "new" foods; but after a while you will level off. I eat a fraction of what I used to eat and can, if I wish, fast for a day or two without any loss of energy; on the contrary, I have more energy. But remember to give yourself time as this may take awhile.

During these coming days many changes will occur in your body for the better, and sometimes it is difficult to understand exactly what is happening. I remember in those early days my body would experience a cleansing crisis (the detoxifying of old poisons) fairly frequently. I would become ill, but three days of eating Bieler's Broth would pull me through very nicely and each crisis would become milder than the one prior. Of course most people do not have the same problems as that and experience only mild symptoms. But it is still important to understand what is happening to your body.

The following are some answers to questions that I have received over the years.

"I am feeling tired even more than usual."

This means that your body is cleansing and your energy is being used for this purpose. It is wise not to increase your food intake (a natural tendency in the past). Try to rest more. This will pass I assure you.

"I am feeling deprived, rather depressed and food is dull."

The reason for this is the same as above. It is difficult in these early days to see your friends and family apparently in good health enjoying themselves eating and drinking anything they desire, while you appear to be eating dull, tasteless food. I can assure you that when your tastebuds return (sometimes for the first time) you will grow to love the new food so much that it will not occur to you to want to change, and the radiant health that is coming your way will more than compensate. Don't worry, the deprived state passes very rapidly.

"When may I start adding new items or some of the foods I was eating in the past?"

It is wise to stay as close as possible to the recommended list of foods for at least three months. At that time you may add a little of the foods eaten previously (such as dairy for example) and your body will let you know if you can or cannot tolerate it. The ideal situation for all of us is to really know what the body needs and can handle. **This is health**. Many times I will receive a telephone call from a client who states that they have included more starch or fruits and discovered that they feel less than well. Of course this obviously means that their body was not yet ready for that change. Just remember that this is a learning and rewarding process, to have this new awareness of your body. "I am experiencing headaches and symptoms similar to a cold, and I have been to see my doctor and he says that I am fine."

Once again it is the same answer, your body is cleansing old toxins. What will make it easier on you is to fast for one to three days on Bieler's Broth or diluted juices. I also found in those early days that it would help if I gave myself an enema.

"I am not satisfied, I am hungry all the time even immediately after eating."

It's that addiction again. This happens almost to everyone in the early days. Your body is going through a lot of cleansing and this creates a gnawing feeling that you will identify as hunger. When this occurs increase your vegetable intake and eat smaller amounts more frequently. Don't worry, this too will pass.

"I am used to having coffee, is there anything that you can recommend to substitute for it?"

In all health food stores you can find a variety of tasteful herbal teas and grain beverages which will work for those who can handle them. It is fun to read about the herbs and to see which ones can fit you and your symptoms. After a while you will not miss coffee.

The stimulants give your body a charge. There is no question that we miss this because we have grown to rely on them to keep the body going, but unfortunately we have deluded ourselves into thinking that this is truly energy. Many people say to me that they must have their early morning coffee or tea to "get them going." As Dr. Bieler put it so well, "it's like flogging a dead horse!" Years ago I was a heavy coffee drinker and I consumed a lot of alcohol and lived on crackers and cheese (now and then I had good meals by accident). People viewed me a person of enormous energy, even when I was very ill, so it was quite interesting for me to observe how little energy I really had after I removed all the props. I soon became aware of how much I cheated myself and Mother Nature for all those years. It was a beautiful experience to be present at my rebirth and to feel the life force and to know what true energy is like.

In conclusion, I would like to remind you that it took many years to bring about the present condition in your body, so do not expect sudden radiant health overnight. But it will come to you in time. We all have the right to be healthy and to experience the full joy of living. It is up to each one of us to live life to the fullest.

● Exercise & Other Self Healing Techniques

Exercise

To create and maintain optimum health requires not only appropriate food choices, but also some form of regular exercise. Energy input (foods) needs to be balanced with energy output (activity).

Most fitness experts now agree that moderate exercise, for at least 20 minutes three times a week is the minimum amount needed to benefit you. Exercise accomplishes many things. It burns calories, and speeds up your metabolism, so you feel more energized, and it relieves stress. It also gives you a sense of well-being and accomplishment, while strengthening and toning muscles, including your most important muscle — your heart!

The exercise you choose should be aerobic, which means during exercise you increase your uptake of oxygen. Your heart rate should rise to about 60 - 70% of your theoretical maximum for at least 20 minutes. To calculate your "target range" first find out your maximum heart rate. Subtract your age from 220. To find your target range, multiply the result by .6 for the minimum, and .7 for the maximum. During exercise take your pulse for 10 seconds and multiply by 6. This lets you know (approximately) if you are within your target heart rate range.

Many forms of exercise will achieve this goal — brisk walking, aerobics, jogging, swimming, roller skating, bicycle riding, dancing, are some of your many options. The important thing is to choose an activity you enjoy. If you enjoy it, you will be more likely to include into your regular schedule.

Other forms of exercise, which are less vigorous, can also benefit the body and mind in slightly different, but overlapping ways. Moving meditations such as Yoga, Tai Chi, and Qi Gong all help to relieve stress, promote balanced energy flow through the body, and help calm and center the mind and spirit. They can be done in addition to aerobic exercise for added benefit (perhaps on alternate days to your aerobic activity!).

When to exercise is a problem many people face. It is best done at a regular time, which you have scheduled just for this purpose. By getting into a routine, it will be easier to be consistent. Many people feel best exercising in the morning because it invigorates them for the day. Others find the evenings better, to wind down from a stressful day. Try both for a while and see what works best for you.

There is no need to go out and train for a marathon. Excessive exercise can lead to injuries, takes too much time, and is not necessary. Whether it is walking, aerobics, dance, yoga or strength training, or working in the garden, remember to choose an activity that is enjoyable and that can be incorporated into your life-style on a continuing basis.

Jin Shin Jyutsu®

Jin Shin Jyutsu® acupressure is a wonderful compliment fo any wellness program. It is an unique self awareness body/mind/spirit harmonizing art as it may be experienced through sessions with a practioner as well as applied as a daily simple self help practice.

To order any of the user friendly self-help books and or practitioner contact phone numbers in your area, call the Jin Shin Jyutsu office at (480) 998-9331, or log on to Jinshinjyutsu.com.

● The Daily Body Feedback Journal

Throughout this book we have given you tools to improve your health, vitality and well-being. Since each of us is biochemically, and energetically unique, one way to find out which things work for us, make us feel and look better, and which things don't, is to keep a daily journal.

By keeping a journal you can learn a lot about how your body responds to different things. The journal is designed so you can keep a record of your daily food intake, your sleep, exercise, and stress patterns, your daily stool and urine output, as well as how you feel emotionally.

Through working with the journal you will become much more familiar with your body and how things affect it. Through this, you will learn what to do and what not to do, what to eat and what not to eat, and how to stay on top of things.

If you ever you begin to feel ill, or just not quite "right," the body feedback journal is a good way to point you in the right direction again. You may find that there is something new affecting you, or something that may not have affected you earlier is affecting you now. As we change, our bodies' needs also change.

The journal can be kept with you and filled out as you go, or you can do the whole day in the evening. Some people find it best to keep the journal with them through the day, for the first few weeks, then switch to morning and evening later on.

After you have a few weeks of journal compiled, you can go back over it and look for correlations. You might find that the day after you eat a particular food, you have gas, or feel constipated. If this happens every time you eat that food, it's a pretty good sign that this is a food you should avoid. Similarly, if you noticed on days that you exercised you had better bowel movements, or felt more energized, you know that is something you should continue to do. Look to both the physical and emotional symptoms as feedback for you to process.

The journals can be a very useful tool for you holistic health practitioner as well. He or she may be able to find patterns in your journal that you may not see right away. They can also gain a better sense of your life-style from your journal.

How to Use the Journal

Use a new page for each day. First note the date, the time you went to bed last night, and the time you rose this morning. You can then figure out how many hours you slept. Women should also note where they are in their menstrual cycle. If a woman is no longer cycling just note the correlations to the lunar cycle, as hormones ebb and flow in all species in relation to lunar cycles.

Your first entry should be about the quality of your sleep. Did you sleep well? Did you wake up? Did you have nightmares? Next, Was it hard to get out of bed? Did you wake up with lots of energy? Then continue on as follows.

Use the journal to record any significant events through the day. Log in the foods you eat, liquids you drink, bowel movements, urination, exercise, a stressful or nervous situation, headaches, gas or other problems, medications or supplements you took (unless you take them every day) and treatments you receive. Note the time, and what you ate, drank and/or did. If it made you feel a particular way, write it down. If you feel a particular way half an hour later, start a new line, write down the time and how you felt.

Stay simple, just recording enough information for you to understand it. If you try to be too detailed, the journal can get to be too much trouble to keep up. It's important to make a commitment to keep the journal for at least one month, as many patterns may not reveal themselves in a shorter time. A sample journal page follows this section. You may copy the sample page for your own use.

Where Do I Start?

If you have read this far and have gone into your kitchen and looked at the ingredient labels of the foods that you have, there is a very good chance that most of the foods that you are eating regularly don't match the recommendations in this book. So where should you start?

Since the body feedback journal will work best if you can start from the basics, I suggest that you do your utmost to eat only the Bieler's vegetables (zucchini, green beans, celery, parsley) and protein (beef, chicken, etc.) for a few days. For most people this is a pleasant experience as they often lose a lot of toxic bloat. Then as you feel like it, begin to add in **one at a time** small amount of grains, starchy vegetables, fruit and/or dairy. If you get a negative reaction, go back to just the vegetables and protein

This is also the procedure that you should follow if you become sick. If you do this your illness will pass in a quarter of the time it would take otherwise. Also as you continue with your new eating plan you will detoxify more and more; and it is very likely that you will get to the point where you almost never get a cold or the flu. I personally have experienced this myself and I have also observed client after client getting to this point of true health.

Body Feedback Journal

Time	Food Eaten (What? How Much?)	Fluid Taken	Effect (physical - emotional)	Activity	Urination	Bowel Movement	Notes

● Simply Delicious Recipes

Quick and Easy Cooking Suggestions

● Borrow a tip from the Asia and wrap an occasional meal in a leaf of lettuce. Spread the lettuce leaf with some low/no sodium mustard and top with sliced or shredded chicken, turkey, salmon, tuna or steamed veggies hot/cold.

● Save cooked leftover veggies and toss with chilled cooked brown rice, shredded lettuce and chilled steamed veggies. Toss lightly with your favorite dressing.

● Steam your favorite veggies with onions or leeks until tender and puree in a blender with a little mirin and herbs for a creamy soup.

● Stretch sauces with chicken stock or lemon juice, not oil or butter.

● Use steamed vegetable water as a base for stocks and sauces.

● Stretch small amounts of fish and chicken by serving on a colorful bed of shredded or julienned cabbage, carrots, zucchini, summer squash, etc., steamed with herbs until tender, crisp.

● Use pureed vegetables to thicken sauces and soups.

● Use lemon juice, not oil, to prevent sticking when cooking pasta.

● Puree carotene rich veggies (orange/yellow colored) with a little cooking water for use in breads and muffins. Best suggestions are: carrots, pumpkin, winter squashes, yams, sweet potatoes.

● Chop your favorite ripe fresh fruits and layer with plain yogurt for a healthy dessert parfait.

● Use a few drops of oil with herbs over baked yams/sweet potatoes/pastas. Toasted sesame oil is particularly tasty!

● Toss 1 Tbls. of sunflower/sesame/pumpkin seeds or pine nuts into your cooked rice for a little extra crunch. Cooked chestnuts are also quite good.

Trimming the Fat (But Not The Flavor!)

Acceptable Cooking Fats (may also be used for non-heated uses):

    Unsalted raw butter
    Olive Oil (extra virgin or virgin only)
    Sesame Oil (toasted or plain)

Acceptable Oils for Non-Heated Uses (Cold-Pressed Only):

Safflower	Avocado	Almond	Hazelnut
Flax	Sunflower	Walnut	

Date all oil when purchased, store in the refrigerator and discard after three months. For optimum health, oil intake should not exceed two Tablespoons daily. Always choose 100% cold expeller pressed oils.

If you choose to include cheeses (raw, rennetless only please) and/or nut butters (unsalted, **no** hydrogenated **fats** or **sugars**) be aware that these are concentrated fats, so adjust your oil intake accordingly.

Most Desirable Cooking Techniques:

Steam	Bake	Grill	
Poach	Stew*	Roast*	
Broil	Water-Saute	Blanch	*incidates not for daily use*

A swipe of oil or butter can be used for flavor in water saute. When blanching, dip veggies in boiling water for a short time.

Stir Fry (for occasional use only) with 1 Tbls. oil, plus chicken/vegetable stock to prevent sticking.

Oil may be tossed into cooked veggies after cooking with a few herbs or spices for flavor. Place oil in small plant mister bottle. Spray on salads, coat a pan for sauteing, or over steamed veggies for a more even coverage with less oil.

Some of the recipes that follow contain spices and condiments that are not for regular daily use or when experiencing less than radiant health. To adapt the recipe, reduce or omit "*the extras*" according to your individual need (see p 20 for the list).

Cereal and Grain Dishes

● **Rice Pilaf**

>1 cup long-grain brown rice
>2 cups water
>2 Tbls. mirin
>2 Tbls. butter
>2 large bay leaves
>1/8 tsp. white pepper
>2 Tbls. chicken stock
>1/2 cup diced green peppers
>1/2 cup diced onions
>1/2 diced mushrooms

Combine ingredients except rice and veggies in 1 1/2 quart saucepan. Bring to a boil. Add rice, cover, turn flame down and simmer for 20 minutes. Stir in vegetables and continue simmering until tender (about 15 minutes). Stir occasionally. Turn off heat and allow to sit covered 10-15 minutes. Fluff with fork, and serve.

● **Millet "Mashed Potatoes"**

>2 1/2 cups water
>1 garlic clove, minced
>1 onion, minced
>2 Tbls. vegetable oil
>1 1/4 cups cauliflower pieces
>1 cup millet
>Freshly ground pepper, to taste

In a large saucepan, saute the garlic and onion in the oil over moderate heat for 5 minutes, until softened. Add the cauliflower, millet and 2 1/2 cups of water. Cover and cook over low heat for 20 minutes.

In a blender or food processor, puree until smooth. Keep warm in a covered saucepan until ready to eat. Serve with Miso Mushroom Gravy (p.61).

● **Home Made Flour** (Millet, Rice, Oat)

To make your own fresh flour from any of the above grains simply grind the grain in a coffee grinder or regular blender until powdered. Any of these flours may be substituted for wheat flour in a recipe. Just make sure to add 1/2 tsp. more of low sodium baking powder than the original recipe calls for.

- **Savory Biscuits**

    2 cups millet/rice/oat flour
    1 1/2 Tbls. low sodium baking powder
    1 Tbls. dill weed
    1/2 tsp. garlic powder
    2 fertile eggs, well beaten
    2 Tbls. unsalted butter

Sift all dry ingredients together. Add eggs and melted butter to form a very stiff dough. If batter is too stiff to handle add a few drops of water. Drop by Tbls. onto a lightly greased baking sheet and bake at 325 degrees for 15 to 20 minutes.

- **French Toast**

    2 slices bread (whole grain)
    2 fertile eggs, well beaten or 2 egg whites & 1 Tbls. water
    2 tsp. cinnamon
    1 tsp. vanilla extract
    1 Tbls. water
    1 Tbls. unsalted butter, melted

Melt butter in a skillet. Blend liquids, eggs, and spices and soak bread until saturated. Brown in skillet on each side and place under broiler to toast briefly. Top with Fruit Compote (see recipe) and/or yogurt.

- **Millet Pilaf**

    2 cups cooked millet
    1 onion, finely chopped
    1 med. tomato, chopped
    1 small apple, peeled and diced
    1 tsp. rosemary
    1/2 tsp. garlic powder or 1 clove, finely chopped
    1/2 tsp. cayenne pepper
    1/2 cup apple juice, unsweetened
    1/2 tsp. curry powder
    1/2 tsp. basil
    2 Tbls. unsalted butter

Melt butter in a skillet and add onions, garlic, herbs, and spices. Saute until onions are transparent. Add apples and juice and saute for an additional 3 to 5 minutes. Stir in millet and tomatoes and cook for 3 to 5 minutes. This may also be used as a delicious stuffing for Cornish game hens, chicken or turkey.

● **Five Minute Breakfast - Grain Custard**

1 large fertile egg
1/4 cup plain or vanilla-pecan amasake or rice/oat milk
1/2 cup cooked grain (brown rice, millet, quinoa, barley, oat groats, kasha, rye berries) or
1/2 cup quick cooking cereal (cream of rye, cream of rice and rye, oatmeal, oat bran)
1/2 tsp. no-sugar vanilla extract
1/2 tsp. cinnamon

Place egg, amasake, vanilla and cinnamon in a blender and whip well. Pour egg mixture into the quick cookinginto a custard-like consistency. Serve immediately topped with fresh fruit, fruit compote, fruit juice sweetened conserves, raisins, or plain.

● **Hot Cereal**

1 cup raw oats/millet/rye/quinoa/amaranth
1 cup water

Cook over low heat until done (rye/oat groats 20-25 minutes, amaranth/millet/quinoa 25-30 minutes).

Toppings: R.W. Knudsen coconut nectar/unsweetened applesauce with cinnamon/chopped fresh fruit/unsweetened fruit jams or butters/amasake/Fruit Compote (see recipe).

● **No Flour Pancakes**

1 cup cooked millet, rice, rye, oats, or mixtures
1 fertile egg
1/4 to 1/2 cup any fruit puree/applesauce

Mix all ingredients in a blender. Drop by spoonful onto a hot nonstick skillet. Cook until lightly browned on both sides. Serve topped with your favorite fruit puree or syrup (a few chopped nuts or seeds may be added to the batter if desired).

- **Summer Pasta Salad**

    2 cups cooked pasta (Kamut, Soba, Rice or Wheat)
    1 - 8 oz. pkg. frozen peas
    2 cups fresh broccoli flowerettes
    3 cloves garlic, minced
    3 Tbls. parsley, finely chopped
    2 Tbls. olive oil
    2 Tbls. mirin
    2 Tbls. fresh basil, finely chopped

Saute broccoli and garlic in olive oil until just tender adding water to prevent sticking. Then add frozen peas and mirin, cover and simmer 5 to 8 minutes. Add parsley and basil and toss briefly with existing veggies. Remove from heat and toss well with pasta. Chill at least one hour and serve cold or at room temperature.

- **Vegetable Couscous**

    1 Tbls. plus 1 tsp. olive oil
    1 med. zucchini quartered lengthwise, thinly sliced
    1 med. yellow squash, quartered lengthwise, thinly sliced
    2 stalks celery, thinly sliced
    5 mushrooms, sliced
    1 small red pepper, diced
    2 Tbls. fresh parsley, finely chopped
    2 cloves garlic, minced, or 3/4 tsp. garlic powder
    2 Tbls. apple cider or rice vinegar
    Juice of one medium lemon and 1 Tbls. water
    1 tsp. cumin powder
    2 cups cooked couscous, quinoa, brown rice, "Riz Cous," or millet.

Coat a large skillet with 1 tsp. olive oil. Place over medium heat and add vegetables and garlic. Saute until tender crisp. Remove from heat and set aside.

In a bowl, mix 1 Tbls. olive oil, cumin, lemon juice, and 1 Tbls. water. Add to the cooked grain of choice and stir to coat well. Fold in sauteed vegetables and serve warm or chilled.

- **Pancakes**

    1 1/2 cups millet/oat/rice flour
    1 tsp. low sodium baking powder
    2 tsp. cinnamon
    1 tsp. vanilla extract
    2 Tbls. melted unsalted butter
    2 fertile eggs or 2 egg whites and 1 Tbls. water
    1/2 cup amasake

Place all ingredients in a blender and blend. Cook pancakes in a lightly greased or nonstick skillet on each side until brown.

Top with Fruit Compote (p.67) and/or yogurt.

- **Stuffed Kabocha Squash**

    2 med. kabocha squash
    3 cups cooked "Lundberg's" wild rice mix
    1/2 cup chopped onion
    1 cup finely chopped celery
    1/2 cup chopped mushrooms
    4 oz. raisins
    4 oz. chopped walnuts or pecans
    2 Tbls. canola oil
    2 tsp. chick-pea miso
    1/2 cup hot water
    1 Tbls. poultry seasoning

Wash kabocha well and place in 1/2" water in an ovenproof pan. Bake at 350 degrees for 45 to 60 minutes or until tender when pierced with a knife. Remove from oven and set aside until cool enough to handle.

Cut a circular slice in the top of the squash and remove all seeds from inside. Saute onion, celery and mushrooms in oil until tender. Add poultry seasoning, raisins, and walnuts and saute briefly until raisins are tender. Remove from heat and mix well with rice. Combine miso with hot water and mix with rice and veggies. Fill each kabocha with the mixture, packing well. Reheat at 350 degrees for 15 to 20 minutes.

Entrees

Note: Red meat is best eaten rare to restore and maintain optimal health. The meat recipes in this section should be considered for occasional use.

- **Chicken Livers in Tomato Sauce**

    *1 lb. **organic** chicken livers*
    1 onion, finely chopped
    2-3 cloves garlic, minced
    2 Tbls. unsalted butter, melted
    1 small can low sodium whole tomatoes/fresh tomatoes chopped
    1 small can low sodium tomato paste
    1/2 cup unsweetened apple juice
    1/2 cup apple cider vinegar
    1/2 tsp. oregano
    1/2 tsp. cayenne pepper
    1 Tbls. basil
    Pepper to taste

Saute onions and garlic in butter 3-5 minutes. Add chicken livers and saute until done. Combine tomato paste with all liquids, herbs and spices, and pour over livers. Add chopped tomatoes and cook 3 to 5 minutes until sauce thickens. Serve over cooked rice or millet, or a bed of steamed julienned vegetables.

- **Salmon with Dill Sauce**

    4 salmon steaks
    1 lemon, plus 1 lemon for garnish
    2 Tbls. dill
    3 Tbls. butter, melted
    2-3 cloves garlic, minced

Combine butter, dill, garlic and juice of one lemon. Broil salmon steaks brushed with mixture and turn over, repeating procedure for other side. Serve topped with remaining dill sauce. Place lemon wedges on the side.

- **Halibut Steak**

    1 halibut steak, 6 oz.
    2 Tbls. lemon juice
    1 Tbls. green onion, sliced
    1/2 cup shredded carrot
    1 Tbls. chopped parsley
    1 tsp. dill weed
    1 small tomato, chopped

Season fish with lemon juice. Reserve tomato and toss all vegetables and herbs together. Spoon on top of fish. Bake, covered at 350 degrees for 30 minutes.

- **Fish en Papillote**

    2 firm-flesh fish fillets, such as cod or halibut
    1 scallion, julienned
    1 lemon, thinly sliced
    1/4 tsp. minced fresh ginger
    Freshly ground black pepper

Preheat oven to 350 degrees. Cut four circles of foil about 10" in diameter, depending on the size of the fish. Place each fillet on one of the circles. Distribute the scallion, lemon, ginger and pepper over the fish. Cover each fillet with another piece of foil, and crimp the edges. Bake fish about 10 minutes per inch of thickness. Serve immediately.

- **Marinated Seafood Steaks**

    Seafood steaks of choice (shark, swordfish, cod, halibut, etc.)
    Marinade (see recipe page 62)

Place seafood steaks in a baking dish with marinade. Marinate 2 or more hours (ideally overnight). Broil or barbecue and serve.

- **Salmon with Apples and Limes**

    2 salmon steaks, 1 1/4 inches thick
    1 apple, sliced into thin 1/2 moons
    1 lime, sliced into thin 1/2 moons
    1 Tbls. butter
    Freshly ground pepper

Saute lime and apple slices in butter until butter is absorbed by fruit (about 5 minutes). Remove lime ends from skillet and rub over salmon, squeezing juice. Sprinkle on pepper. Broil salmon 7 minutes per side. Serve immediately topped with sauteed fruit.

- **Stir Fried Shrimp**

    1 1/2 Tbls. sesame oil
    10 large shrimp, cleaned
    1/4 cup green peppers and onion
    1/4 cup snow peas
    1/4 cup red cabbage, chopped

Heat oil in small skillet. Add shrimp and stir-fry for 2 minutes. Add remaining ingredients and cook 3 more minutes.

● Poached Salmon

> *5 oz. salmon steak*
> *1/4 cup chicken broth*
> *2 Tbls. mirin*
> *2 Tbls. water*
> *1 tsp. dijon mustard*

Simmer salmon covered in broth and mirin for 8 to 10 minutes. Remove fish, boil broth until reduced slightly. Mix water, mustard and arrowroot and add to broth. Cook until thickened. Serve on a bed of steamed julienned vegetables topped with sauce.

● Fluffy Omelette

> *3 eggs, separated*
> *1/2 tsp. basil*
> *1 tsp. dijon mustard*
> *2 Tbls. unsalted butter*

Whip egg whites until very stiff in a chilled bowl. Beat egg yolks in a separate bowl with all herbs and spices. Fold yolk mixture carefully into egg whites. Melt butter in a skillet and add egg mixture. Cook over low heat until bottom is lightly browned when edge is lifted with a fork. Place under broiler until lightly browned.

Fill with curried or sauteed vegetables, tomato sauce, Italian chicken livers, etc. Fold and turn onto plate. Top as desired.

● Crunchy Sole

> *1 lb. sole*
> *1 zucchini, thinly sliced*
> *1/4 cup walnuts, chopped, or crushed rice cakes*
> *1 Tbls. walnut oil*
> *1/2 tsp. dried or 1 tsp. fresh tarragon*
> *Lemon and pepper to taste*

Line baking dish with foil, place sole on half. Top with zucchini and walnuts. Sprinkle with walnut oil and oregano. Add lemon and pepper to taste. Bring other half of foil over the top and seal edges. Prick holes in foil with a fork. Bake at 325 for 25 minutes.

- **Stuffed Cornish Game Hens**

    2 organic ethically-raised cornish game hens
    1 Millet Pilaf (see recipe page 35)
    1 cup unsweetened apple juice

Place game hens stuffed with millet recipe in foil lined baking dish and bake at 350 degrees for 30 to 40 minutes. Baste frequently with apple juice. Bake last 10 minutes at 475 to brown hens.

- **Sole Royal**

    1/2 lb. sole fillets
    3 Tbls. lemon juice
    1 tsp. apple concentrate
    1/2 tsp. dill weed
    1 Tbls. butter
    1 tsp. chopped parsley

Season fish with 1 Tbls. lemon juice. Heat slowly remaining ingredients except parsley. Saute fish in butter, 1 1/2 minutes per side. Serve fish with sauce and parsley garnish.

- **Tuna with Dill Sauce**

    2 cups cauliflower, broken into small pieces
    4 crookneck yellow squash in uniform chunks
    1/2 small onion
    2-3 cloves garlic
    1 cup no salt chicken stock
    2 Tbls. mirin
    1 Large can Tuna

Simmer until tender. Puree in blender until very smooth with:

   1 Tbls. dijon mustard
   1 Tbls. dill weed

Place back in saucepan with 1 large can flaked tuna and heat. Serve on a bed of julienned steamed zucchini.

- **Lemon Chicken**

    4 organic ethically-raised boneless chicken breasts
    1 lemon, thinly sliced
    1 Tbls. rosemary
    2 tsp. garlic powder

In a foil lined baking dish arrange chicken breasts on top of lemon slices and sprinkle with spice mixture. Bake at 425 degrees for 20 to 25 minutes.

- **Italian Chicken**

    6 organic ethically-raised chicken breasts
    2 zucchini, sliced
    2 fluted squash, sliced
    2 tomatoes, chopped
    1 onion, chopped
    1/2 lb. sliced mushrooms
    1 cup unsweetened apple juice
    1/2 cup apple cider vinegar
    1 tsp. garlic powder
    1/2 tsp. cayenne pepper
    1/2 tsp. rosemary
    1/2 tsp. oregano
    1 tsp. arrowroot
    1/2 tsp. basil

Place chicken breasts on top of veggie mixture in a foil lined baking dish. Combine all herbs, spices and liquids and pour over chicken. Bake uncovered at 375 degrees for 30 to 40 minutes.

- **Non-Dairy Zucchini Quiche**

    1 whole wheat pie shell
    1 leek or yellow onion, sliced
    2 zucchini diced
    2 Tbls. parsley, finely chopped
    1 Tbls. olive oil (extra-virgin)
    1/2 tsp. oregano
    1/4 tsp. black pepper
    1/2 tsp. basil
    1 Tbls. mirin
    3 fertile eggs, beaten + 1 tsp. dijon mustard

Saute vegetables in oil until tender and add mirin/herbs. Transfer veggies to pie shell. Pour egg mixture over veggies and bake at 350 for 45 to 50 minutes or until crust is done.

- **Quick Moo-Shu Veggie Wraps**

    2 to 4 "Tannour" bread <u>or</u> 2 to 4 sheets nori
    1/2 cup finely sliced celery
    1 cup finely shredded romaine lettuce
    1/4 cup peas
    1/4 cup finely grated carrots
    1 Tbls. sesame oil
    1 tsp. mirin
    1 Tbls. tamari
    1/4 cup water
    1/2 cup finely shredded red cabbage
    1/2 cup finely shredded white cabbage
    1/4 cup finely chopped mushrooms
    1 clove garlic, minced, <u>or</u> 1/4 cup sliced scallions
    1/4 cup cubed tofu (mirin/tamari marinade optional)

Saute celery, garlic/scallions, peas, carrots, and mushrooms in oil until tender. Add water, then cabbage and romaine until barely tender. Add tofu, mirin and tamari. Serve immediately rolled in "Tannour" bread or nori seaweed sheets.

- **Lamb/Veal chops in Balsamic Sauce**

    4 ethically-raised veal or lean lamb chops
    1 cup chicken stock
    1 Tbls. olive oil
    1/2 Tbls. garlic, minced
    1/4 cup balsamic vinegar
    1 Tbls. parsley, finely chopped
    1 Tbls. fresh mint, finely chopped

In a saucepan, boil stock to reduce volume by half, then set aside.

In a small skillet saute garlic in olive oil until golden brown. Add in reduced chicken stock and vinegar. Reduce volume by half again, over high heat. Add in parsley and mint and set aside.

Broil lamb/veal chops on each side until done to individual taste. Transfer to a heated platter surrounding edges with steamed vegetable of choice and spoon sauce over meat. Serve immediately.

● Chicken Ala King

> 2 to 4 organic ethically-raised chicken breasts
> 50/50 cauliflower and crook neck yellow squash
> 2 cloves garlic
> 1 cup chicken stock <u>or</u> 6 cubes frozen stock
> 2 Tbls. mirin

Simmer all ingredients in a covered saucepan until tender. Place in a blender with:

> 1/2 tsp. poultry herb mix
> 1 tsp. dill
> 1 Tbls. dijon style mustard

Puree until very smooth. Pour back into saucepan and fold in cubed or shredded cooked meat from 2 to 4 chicken breasts. Serve over lightly steamed julienned zucchini. Garnish with paprika.

● Chicken with Artichoke Heart

> 4 boneless, skinless, organic, ethically-raised chicken breasts, pounded thinly
> 2 cups homemade chicken broth, <u>or</u> 10 cubes frozen chicken broth
> 2 cloves garlic, minced
> 1/2 medium onion, thinly sliced
> 2 stalks celery, thinly sliced
> 2 Tbls. olive oil
> 2 Tbls. mirin
> 3 Tbls. parsley, finely chopped
> 2 pkgs. frozen artichoke hearts

Saute garlic, onions, and celery in olive oil until translucent. Add chicken breasts and brown on both sides. Add mirin and broth to pan, cover, and simmer 20 to 25 minutes.

Add artichoke hearts and simmer covered 5 to 8 more minutes. Remove cover, add parsley and reduce pan juices to desired consistency over high heat. Serve immediately.

- **Potted Chicken**

    1 whole organic ethically-raised chicken, cut into parts and skinned (remove all visible fat)
    2 cups chicken stock (See recipe P. 33)
    3 Tbls. mirin
    1/4 tsp. pepper
    1 bay leaf
    2 cloves garlic, minced
    4 carrots, diced
    2 stalks celery, diced
    1/2 onion, chopped coarsely
    2 Tbls. parsley, chopped

Simmer covered 35 minutes then add:

   2 cups diced zucchini/crook neck yellow squash

Cook covered 8 to 10 minutes.

- **Chicken Livers in Brown Sauce**

    *3/4 lb. **organic** ethically raised chicken livers*
    2 tsp. olive oil
    2 Tbls. mirin
    1 tsp. "Robbie's" worcestershire sauce
    1/2 cup chicken stock

Saute livers in oil until lightly browned. Add remaining ingredients and simmer covered for 10-12 minutes. Add 1 1/2 cups "White Sauce" (see recipe page 66).

   1/2 tsp. garlic powder
   1/2 tsp. "Parsley Patch" seafood blend
   1/4 tsp. pepper

Fold above into the chicken liver mixture and serve over a bed of steamed julienned vegetables.

- **Carolyn's Tuna in Cream Sauce**

    50/50 cauliflower and crook neck yellow squash sliced into uniform pieces
    1 can flaked white meat tuna, 8 oz.
    1 small yellow onion, skinned
    2 cloves garlic, peeled
    3 Tbls. fresh cilantro chopped coarsely
    1 Tbls. fresh dill chopped coarsely
    2 Tbls. mirin
    1 Tbls. dijon style mustard

Simmer all ingredients in covered saucepan until tender. Place in blender with /mustard, puree until very smooth. Return to saucepan, add tuna. Serve on bed of steamed julienned carrots/zucchini.

- **Tofu Burgers**

    4 oz. well drained tofu (Chinese style)
    1 Tbls. miso (chick-pea is best)
    1 Tbls. chopped scallions
    1 tsp. mirin
    1 tsp. oil

Crumble tofu and add miso and mirin until well mixed. Fold in scallions. Form into a patty and saute in oil preferably in a nonstick skillet. Best served open faced on a rice cake.

- **Asparagus with Poached Eggs in Vinegarette**

    1 lb. asparagus   *Whisk Vinegarette:*
    2 to 4 fertile eggs   *4 Tbls. lemon juice*
        2 Tbls. walnut/almond oil
        1/2 tsp. dijon mustard

Poach eggs and serve warm on top of chilled asparagus. Spoon Vinegarette over eggs and asparagus.

- **Basil Chicken**

    4 pounded, organic, ethically-raised, boneless, skinless, chicken breasts, marinated overnight in:
    1/4 cup finely chopped parsley
    1/4 cup finely chopped basil
    3 cloves finely minced garlic
    1/2 tsp. "Parsley Patch" Italian blend herb mix
    3/4 cup chicken stock
    3 Tbls. mirin
    2 Tbls. "Robbie's" worcestershire

Saute chicken on each side 3-5 minutes in a small amount of marinade until tender. Add remaining marinade and steam covered 10-15 minutes. Serve on a bed of chopped steamed broccoli/escarole.

- **Braised Veal Chops with Cabbage**

    2 ethically raised veal chops (rib best)
    2 Tbls. butter
    1 cup chicken stock
    3 Tbls. mirin
    2 Tbls. "Robbie's" worcestershire sauce
    2 cloves garlic, minced
    2 Tbls. parsley, finely chopped
    2 stalks celery, finely chopped
    2 cups white cabbage, shredded

Saute veal chops, garlic, and celery in butter until lightly browned on each side. Add stock, mirin, worcestershire, parsley, and celery and simmer covered over low heat 30 minutes. Add cabbage and cook covered 10 more minutes.

- **Veal Chops Calabres**

    2 ethically raised veal Rib/Loin chops
    2 Tbls. olive oil
    4 cloves garlic, chopped
    2 Tbls. lemon juice
    1 cup chicken stock
    1 green bell pepper, thinly sliced
    1 red bell pepper, thinly sliced
    1/2 onion, sliced thinly in half moons

Saute veal chops in oil on both sides until lightly browned. Remove to a plate and add garlic, all liquids and veggies. Cook until tender. Reduce liquids over high heat then add the chops to heat thoroughly.

- **Meat Loaf**

    1/4 cup parsley, finely chopped
    1-2 med. zucchini, finely chopped
    2 cloves garlic, finely chopped
    2 stalks celery, finely chopped
    2 crook neck yellow squash, finely chopped
    1/2 med. onion
    2 Tbls. mirin
    1 Tbls. "Robbies" worchestershire sauce
    Black pepper to taste
    1 lb. ethically raised veal, ground or ground organic chicken

Mix all ingredients well by hand. Form into a loaf shape and bake uncovered at 350 degrees for 45 to 50 minutes.

Soups

• Minestrone Soup

>   *1 Tbls. safflower oil*
>   *1 small onion*
>   *1 large carrot, sliced*
>   *1 stalk celery, chopped*
>   *1 fresh tomato, chopped*
>   *1 Tbls. tomato paste*
>   *1/4 cup cooked beans*
>   *3 cups chicken broth*
>   *2 cups chopped zucchini/yellow squash/cauliflower/broccoli*
>   *1/4 tsp. celery seed*
>   *1/4 tsp. oregano*
>   *1/4 tsp. basil*
>   *Pepper to taste*
>   *1/2 cup cooked macaroni (whole wheat)*

Heat oil in a large stock pot. Saute onion slowly until tender. Add carrots and celery and cook until golden brown. Add tomato and tomato paste. Stir to blend with other ingredients. Add beans and stir slowly. Add chicken broth, herbs and seasoning. Simmer covered for about 20 minutes, or until vegetables are tender. Add cooked macaroni and cook 3 to 5 more minutes. Serve hot.

• Cream of Cauliflower

>   *1/2 med. cauliflower, sliced*
>   *1 leek, sliced*
>   *2 yellow crook neck squash, sliced*
>   *1 clove garlic*
>   *1/4 tsp. marjoram*
>   *1 tsp. butter or oil*
>   *Water or chicken stock to barely cover vegetables*

Place all ingredients in a soup pot and simmer covered for 15 to 20 minutes or until tender. Puree in blender and serve hot.

● Ginger Carrot Bisque

3 carrots, sliced
2 stalks celery, sliced
2 small zucchini, sliced
2 cloves garlic
1/2 tsp. grated ginger root
1 cup chicken/vegetable stock

Simmer all ingredients in a covered pot for 20 to 25 minutes. Puree in blender and serve hot or chilled.

● Winter Squash Bisque

2 cups cubed cooked winter squash (acorn, banana, butternut, buttercup, kabocha, Hokkaido)
1/2 small onion <u>or</u> 1 leek sliced
Grated ginger to taste
1 cup water/chicken/vegetable stock

Simmer all ingredients in a pot covered for 20 to 25 minutes. Puree in a blender and serve hot.

● Country Pottage

1 potato, cubed
1 carrot, sliced
1 leek, sliced
1 clove garlic
1 tsp. butter or oil
1 bay leaf
Water/chicken stock to cover

Simmer all ingredients in a covered pot for 20 to 25 minutes. Remove bay leaf and puree in blender. Serve hot.

● **Curried Carrot Soup with Chives**

1 Tbls. unsalted butter
1/4 peeled onion, coarsely chopped
4 carrots, peeled and coarsely chopped
2 yellow squash, chopped
1 celery stalk, coarsely chopped
1/2 clove garlic, minced
3 Tbls. curry powder
3 cups chicken stock
Freshly ground white pepper to taste
Vegetable seasoning to taste

Garnish: 2 Tbls. chopped chives

In a large pot, melt butter, add chopped vegetables and garlic, and saute 4 minutes, stirring over medium heat. Add curry powder and cook 3 minutes more, stirring constantly. Do not allow curry to burn. Add chicken stock, turn up heat to high, and bring to a boil. Lower heat and simmer mixture, uncovered, for 30 minutes. Puree mixture in a blender or food processor and serve hot.

●● **"Bieler's" Soup**

1 lb. fresh or frozen whole green beans
2 to 4 stalks celery sliced with strings removed (optional)
4 to 6 med. sliced zucchini sliced
1 handful parsley tops (no stems)

Fill a large pot with 1/3 water and add all ingredients. Cover and cook in rapidly boiling water for 15-18 minutes or until the vegetables are fork tender. Then place all ingredients in blender and <u>puree in batches until smooth</u>. Season with any of your favorite herbs, i.e., paprika, oregano, garlic, lemon or basil. Serve hot or cold. DO NOT ADD SALT.

- **Quick Minestrone**

    1/2 cup pasta sauce
    1 1/2 cups chicken stock
    1 tsp. oregano
    1 tsp. basil
    1/4 tsp. black pepper
    1 pinch red pepper
    1 cup cooked beans (optional)
    2 carrots, sliced
    1 onion, chopped
    2 stalks celery, sliced
    3 to 4 zucchini or yellow squash, sliced
    1 cup cooked leftover rice
    2-3 Tbls. chopped parsley

Place all ingredients in a large soup pot. Simmer over low-medium heat until veggies are just tender. Great to use with leftover rice/beans.

- **Meatball Soup**

    3/4 pound ground organic ethically raised veal/chicken/or turkey
    Pepper/garlic/basil to taste
    1 1/2 Tbls. "Robbie's" worcestershire sauce

Mix all above ingredients well by hand, and form into walnut size balls. Place in the bottom of a large covered saucepan, add:

    2 cups of shredded white cabbage
    2 cups of julienned crook neck yellow squash.
    1/2 cups of chicken stock or 6 cubes frozen stock
    4 Tbls. mirin
    1/2 tsp. garlic powder (optional)
    1 1/2 Tbls. "Robbie's" worcestershire sauce
    Pepper to taste

Place all ingredients in a large covered saucepan, bring to a boil, then simmer over medium-low heat for 25 to 30 minutes.

- **Cream of Celery**

    2 1/2 cups cauliflower broken into uniform pieces
    3 stalks of celery (strings removed) sliced
    2 cloves of garlic, peeled (optional)
    1 cup or 6 cubes of frozen chicken stock
    3 Tbls. mirin

Simmer all ingredients in a large covered saucepan until tender. Place in a blender and puree until very smooth.

- **Zucchini Milanese Soup**

    3 to 4 medium zucchini, sliced
    2 cups of cauliflower sliced
    2 cloves of garlic, peeled
    1 1/2 cups of chicken stock, <u>or</u> 6 cubes of frozen chicken stock
    1 Tbls. of "Parsley Patch" Italian herb seasoning
    2 Tbls. mirin
    Pepper to taste

Simmer all ingredients in a covered saucepan until tender. Place in a blender and puree until very smooth

- **Chunky Chicken Soup**

    Shredded chicken from 4 cooked organic, ethically-raised chicken breasts
    1 cup julienned zucchini
    1/2 cup of thinly sliced celery
    1/2 yellow onion, thinly sliced
    1 cup julienned crook neck yellow squash
    2 cups chicken stock <u>or</u> 8 cubes frozen stock
    3 Tbls. mirin
    1/2 tsp. garlic powder
    Pepper to taste

Simmer ingredients in large covered saucepan 20 to 25 minutes.

- **Mock French Onion Soup**

    2 yellow onions, thinly sliced
    2 cloves garlic minced
    2 cups chicken/vegetable stock
    1 or 2 squares mochi cubed

Place all ingredients except mochi in a pot and simmer for 20 to 25 minutes. Add mochi and cook stirring frequently until mochi "melts." Serve immediately.

- **Zucchini Consomme**

    1 tsp. mirin
    1/2 tsp. thyme
    1/2 tsp. basil
    2 cups homemade or low-sodium chicken broth
    2 cups shredded zucchini

Combine in saucepan, bring to boil, simmer 20 min. Serve hot.

- **Quick Basic Chicken Stock**

    4 skinless, organic, ethically-raised chicken breasts
    4 to 5 cups water
    3 Tbls. mirin
    2 cloves garlic, peeled
    1 small yellow onion, peeled
    1 handful of parsley
    2 stalks of celery
    1 carrot, peeled
    Pepper to taste
    1 bay leaf

Place ingredients in large covered stock pot, boil. Lower the heat and simmer for 1 1/2 hours. Remove chicken breasts and save for another recipe (See Chicken a la King p.44, and Chunky Chicken Soup, p.52). Strain liquid to be used fresh or pour into ice cube trays. Freeze and pop out into freezer bags. Store ice cubes in freezer for future use.

● Curried Zucchini Soup

Oil from mister
1 med. onion, chopped
2 med. carrots, chopped
4 celery stalks, chopped
4 to 6 zucchini, sliced
1 tsp. curry powder, or to taste
1 1/2 cups chicken stock
Salt-free seasoning to taste

Mist a medium soup pot with oil. Heat over medium heat. Add onion, carrots, celery, and 1 to 2 Tbls. chicken stock, and saute until onions are soft. Add remaining ingredients. Bring to a boil, cover, reduce heat to low and simmer until vegetables are tender-crisp, about 10 to 15 minutes. Strain vegetables and set broth aside. Place vegetables in food processor or blender. Puree until smooth; add broth until soup reaches desired consistency. Return puree to soup pot. Adjust seasonings. Heat over low heat.

Salads

• Salad Ideas

Sliced raw zucchini, cucumber, cabbage, cauliflower, watercress, carrots, jicama, Jerusalem artichokes, sprouts, parsley, and yellow squash are great additions to the normal lettuce salad. Use any of the salad dressing recipes listed or your own favorites (go easy on the oil).

• Marinated Salad

> *1 lb. green beans*
> *2 cups cauliflower broken into large pieces*
> *1 onion, finely chopped*
> *3 Tbls. finely chopped parsley*
> *1 cucumber, thinly sliced*
> *1 cup Seafood/Veggie Marinade (see recipe page 62)*

Steam green beans and cauliflower until just tender. Place all ingredients in a bowl and toss. Chill well. Before serving, toss again.

• Bean Salad

> *1 cup steamed green beans*
> *1/2 cup cooked garbanzo beans or pinto beans*
> *1/2 cup sliced leek*

• Dressing

> *2 Tbls. chick pea miso*
> *Juice of 1 lemon*
> *1/2 tsp. mustard*

Mix dressing well and fold in veggies and beans. Chill well and serve.

- **Cabbage Salad**

    2 cups finely sliced red cabbage
    2 cups finely sliced green cabbage
    1/2 cup grated carrots
    1/2 cup finely chopped apples
    1 cup Seafood/Veggie Marinade (see recipe page 62)

Place all ingredients in a bowl, toss, and chill until ready to serve.

- **Quick Tabouli Bean Salad**

    1 pkg. "Cedar Lane" pre-prepared no salt tabouli
    1 can garbanzos, rinsed well and drained
    2 stalks celery, diced
    4 to 6 radishes, diced
    1 to 2 tomatoes, cubed
    1 cucumber, diced and peeled

Gently fold veggies and beans into tabouli mixture. Serve on a bed of lettuce or in a lettuce lined pita

Vegetables

- **Baked Cinnamon Yams**

    2 large yams, washed and scrubbed
    2 Tbls. unsalted melted butter
    1 Tbls. cinnamon
    1/2 tsp. ginger powder
    1/2 tsp. pepper

Mix all ingredients except yams well. Bake yams in foil at 400 degrees until done (usually 30 to 45 minutes). Remove from foil, slice open and drizzle with butter mixture.

- **Chinese Stirfry**

    1/2 lb. asparagus, sliced diagonally
    1/2 cup bamboo shoots
    1/2 cup bean sprouts
    3 green onions, sliced
    1/2 lb. Chinese pea pods
    1 zucchini, thinly sliced
    3 cloves garlic, finely chopped
    6-8 water chestnuts
    1 Tbls. sesame oil
    1/2 tsp. ginger, grated
    1/2 cup unsweetened apple juice
    1/2 tsp. curry powder
    1/2 cup chicken stock

Place onions, garlic, herbs, and spices in a large skillet and add oil and chicken stock. Saute at high heat for 3 to 5 minutes. Add apple juice and remaining ingredients, cook on high heat stirring occasionally for 5 to 8 minutes or until veggies reach desired crispness..

- **Curried Sweet Potatoes**

    3 to 4 sweet potatoes, cubed
    1/2 cup Curry Sauce (see recipe, page 61)

Steam sweet potatoes 10 to 15 minutes. Mash and blend with Curry Sauce. Pour into foil lined baking dish and bake at 375 degrees for 15 to 20 minutes.

- **Pepper and Zucchini Saute**

    1/2 onion, thinly sliced
    2 zucchini, thinly sliced
    1 red or green pepper, sliced
    2 to 3 cloves garlic, finely chopped
    1/2 tsp. basil
    1/2 tsp. pepper
    1 Tbls. olive oil
    2 Tbls. chicken stock
    1/2 tsp. rosemary

Saute onion, garlic, herbs, and spices in oil and chicken stock mixture. Add zucchini and pepper and cook covered an additional 5 to 8 minutes.

- **Breakfast Zucchini Saute**

    1 onion, finely chopped
    3 zucchini, grated
    1 clove garlic, finely chopped
    1/2 tsp. basil
    1/2 tsp. cayenne pepper
    1/2 cup chicken stock
    2 Tbls. unsalted butter
    3 fertile eggs, beaten well

Melt butter in skillet, add onion, garlic. Saute until tender. Add zucchini, basil, cayenne, and chicken stock. Saute until well done. Pour eggs over top and cook without stirring until set.

- Yam Souffle #1

    2 fertile egg whites
    1 large yam, cooked and mashed
    1 Tbls. apple juice concentrate
    1/2 tsp. cinnamon

Beat egg whites until very stiff. In a food processor, combine yam, juice, cinnamon, and blend until smooth. Gently fold in egg whites. Pour into a heatproof souffle dish and bake at 375 degrees for 25 to 30 minutes. Serve immediately.

● **Yam Souffle #2**

>   2 fertile egg whites
>   1 large yam, cooked and mashed
>   1 Tbls. low sodium tamari
>   1/2 tsp. ground ginger
>   1 Tbls. apple juice

● **Spicy Squash**

>   2 Tbls. vegetable oil
>   1 med. onion, chopped
>   2 garlic cloves, minced
>   1/2 tsp. minced fresh ginger
>   1/2 tsp. dry hot red pepper flakes
>   1/2 cup chicken stock
>   1/4 cup turmeric
>   1 Tbls. apple juice concentrate
>   1 lb. butternut squash, peeled and cut into 1/2 inch cubes

Place the oil in a large skillet over moderate heat. Cook the onion and garlic until tender. Stir in the ginger, hot pepper, turmeric, apple juice and 1/2 cup chicken stock. Add the squash cubes and cook, stirring for 5 minutes. Cover, reduce the heat to low, and cook for 10 minutes longer, until the squash is soft but still firm.

● **Ratatoulle with Rosemary**

>   1 med. zucchini, sliced
>   1 med. summer squash, sliced
>   1 med. eggplant, cubed
>   3 tomatoes, chopped
>   1 red pepper, chopped
>   1 clove garlic, finely minced
>   1 onion, finely chopped
>   2 Tbls. vegetable oil
>   1/4 tsp. pepper
>   1 Tbls. fresh basil, finely minced
>   1 tsp. fresh rosemary, finely chopped
>   1 tsp. fresh parsley, finely chopped

In a skillet, heat the oil and saute the onion and garlic until tender. Put the vegetables, herbs, salt and pepper into a casserole dish. Pour the onion over the vegetables and toss well. Cover the casserole and bake in a preheated 350 degrees oven for 45 minutes. Serve hot or cold.

- **Eggplant - Zucchini Salad**

    2 small eggplants, about 1/2 lb each
    3 med. red bell peppers
    2 med. zucchini diced into 1" pieces
    3 Tbls. olive oil
    2 Tbls. lemon juice
    1/2 tsp. oregano
    1 garlic clove, minced
    2 Tbls. fresh parsley, chopped

Broil eggplants and peppers for 5 to 7 minutes on each side or until slightly charred. Cool. Remove skin. Dice eggplants into 1" pieces. Seed red peppers and cut into strips. Steam vegetable until tender crisp. In a bowl combine olive oil, lemon juice, oregano, garlic and parsley. Chill vegetables in marinade at least 2 hours.

- **Lemon Summer Squash**

    1 clove garlic, minced
    2 Tbls. Fresh parsley, minced
    1 tsp. grated lemon peel
    2 med. zucchini, julienned
    2 med. yellow squash, julienned
    1/2 cup chicken broth
    1/8 tsp. pepper

Saute yellow squash and zucchini in 3 Tbls. chicken broth until just tender, add remaining broth, simmer covered 5 to 8 minutes. Stir in garlic, lemon peel and parsley and cook uncovered 3 to 5 more minutes. Serve hot, cold or at room temperature.

- **Balsamic Zucchini**

    4 med. zucchini sliced into thin 1/2 moons
    1 med shallot, minced
    2 Tbls. olive oil
    1 Tbls. balsamic vinegar
    2 Tbls. fresh mint, finely chopped
    Pepper to taste

Saute shallot and zucchini in olive oil until tender crisp (adding water or broth if necessary to prevent sticking). Add vinegar, mint and pepper. Allow to stand for at least 15 minutes in order for flavors to blend and deepen. Serve at room temperature.

Beat egg whites until very stiff. In a food processor, combine yam, juice, ginger and tamari and blend until smooth. Gently fold in egg whites. Pour into a heatproof souffle dish and bake at 375 degrees for 25 to 30 minutes. Serve immediately.

- **Blister Potatoes**

    2 large potatoes

Preheat oven to 350 degrees. Wash potatoes but do not peel. Slice into 1/4 inch circles. Place directly on a nonstick cookie sheet. Bake for 30 minutes or until potatoes are brown and have a "blister" on top. Remove from oven carefully with a spatula. Brush with **Garlic Butter Sauce:**

    2 Tbls. butter
    1/2 tsp. garlic powder

In a small saucepan, melt butter with garlic powder.

- **Marinated Fresh Vegetables with Fennel**

    1 Tbls. oil
    3 Tbls. water
    1 Tbls. apple cider vinegar
    1/2 tsp. oregano
    1/2 tsp. thyme
    1 Tbls. parsley
    6 peppercorns
    1 or 2 peeled garlic cloves (optional)
    1/8 tsp. fennel seeds
    Pinch of celery seeds and salt (optional)
    2 to 3 cups fresh artichoke hearts, carrots, cauliflower, mushrooms, cucumbers, peppers, green beans in season.

In a saucepan combine oil, water, and vinegar. Bring to a boil, add herbs, and cook slowly for about 5 minutes. Remove from heat and cool. Steam vegetables until tender. Store marinade and vegetables together in refrigerator overnight. Serve cold.

Sauces/Spreads/Dips/Dressing

• Vinegarette Dressing

1 tsp. dijon-style mustard
1 tsp. chick pea miso
1 Tbls. extra-virgin olive oil
1/2 tsp. basil
1/8 tsp. black pepper
1 clove crushed garlic
2 Tbls. brown rice vinegar
1 Tbls. apple juice concentrate
1 Tbls. water with 1/2 tsp. mirin

Mix all ingredients well and chill until ready to use.

• Miso Mushroom Gravy

1 Tbls. sesame oil
1 lb. mushrooms, sliced
1 onion, thinly sliced
1 Tbls. arrowroot
1 Tbls. natural worcestershire sauce (optional)
1 1/2 cups water
1 Tbls. tamari
1 Tbls. miso
Freshly ground pepper, to taste

In a large saucepan, cook mushrooms and onions in the sesame oil over moderately low heat for 10 minutes, until the mushrooms release their juices. Dissolve the arrowroot in the tamari, miso, and worcestershire, stir into mushroom mixture. Add 1 1/2 cups water, increase the heat to moderate and cook for 15 minutes, stirring occasionally, until thickened. Season as desired.

- **Curry Sauce**

    2 Tbls. curry powder
    1/2 cup water
    1/2 cup unsweetened apple juice
    1 onion, quartered
    3 garlic cloves
    1/2 tsp. cumin
    1/2 tsp. tumeric
    1 tsp. freshly grated ginger

Steam onion and garlic 3 to 5 minutes. Place in a saucepan and add remaining ingredients. Simmer 3 to 5 minutes. Puree mixture in a blender. This sauce is delicious over steamed veggies, over sauteed chicken slices and veggies, scrambled eggs, broiled lamb or chicken.

- **Seafood/Veggie Marinade**

    1/3 cup apple juice concentrate
    1/2 cup apple cider vinegar
    1 glove garlic crushed
    1 tsp. basil
    3/4 tsp. dijon-style mustard
    1/8 tsp. ground white pepper

Combine and use as a marinade for any seafood or veggie dish.

- **Fresh Quick Herb Dip**

    2 cups low-fat yogurt
    2 Tbls. chopped fresh parsley
    1 Tbls. fresh dill weed
    1 tsp. chopped fresh chives
    1 tsp. fresh marjoram
    Garlic (optional)

Blend herbs with yogurt and chill. Serve with raw vegetables.

- **Low-Calorie Pseudo Pesto**

    1 1/2 cups loosely packed fresh basil leaves
    1/2 cup loosely flat-leaf (Italian) parsley leaves
    2 Tbls. fresh lemon juice with ° cup water
    2 Tbls. Olive oil
    2 tsp. freshly ground black pepper

In a food processor fitted with the steel blade, process basil and parsley. In a thin stream, as if making a mayonnaise, add the lemon juice and 3/4 cup water. Pepper sparingly. Let sit for at least 1/2 hour before serving. (Keeps 3 to 4 days refrigerated.)

- **Special Sour Cream**

    1 cup water
    1/8 tsp. sea salt
    4 oz. tofu
    1 layer of 12" X 12" cheesecloth
    1/2 Tbls. lemon juice

Bring water to a boil. Add salt. Drop in tofu and return water to boil. Remove pan from heat and allow to sit for three minutes. Remove tofu with a slotted spoon and place in center of cheesecloth. Pull four corners of cheesecloth up, twist tight, and squeeze all excess water from tofu. Place tofu, lemon juice, and salt into a blender or food processor and puree until smooth. Yields about 1/2 cup. Use whenever sour cream is called for.

- **Quick Catsup**

    2 small cans low sodium tomato paste
    1/2 cup unsweetened apple juice
    1/2 cup apple cider vinegar
    1/2 tsp. oregano
    1 to 2 dashes cayenne pepper

Place all ingredients in a saucepan and simmer 3 to 5 minutes. Chill until ready to use.

- **Herb Blend**

    1 tsp. each: *dried basil*
    marjoram
    thyme
    oregano
    parsley
    summer savor
    ground cloves
    mace
    black pepper
    1/4 tsp. each: *ground nutmeg*
    cayenne pepper

Combine herbs in a jar with a tight-fitting lid. Store in a cool place up to six months. Use as a seasoning for meats and vegetables.

- **Sour Cream Potato Topping**

    1/2 cup yogurt
    1/4 cup chopped parsley
    Paprika to taste 1 Tbls. lemon juice

Fold yogurt, parsley, and lemon juice together and top a baked potato. Sprinkle with paprika and serve.

- **Baked Potato Topping**

    1/2 bell pepper, diced
    1 Tbls. olive oil
    3 sliced mushrooms
    1/2 small onion, minced
    1 clove garlic, minced
    1 Tbls. chopped parsley
    Herbs of choice to taste (basil, rosemary, tarragon)

Saute onions and garlic until transparent. Add remaining ingredients and cook slowly over low heat until done. Additional water may be added to prevent sticking at any time. Serve over baked potato with steamed greens or a salad.

- **Tomato Sauce**

    10 oz. can low sodium tomatoes, whole
    1 small can low sodium tomato paste
    1/2 cup unsweetened apple juice
    1/2 cup water
    1/2 tsp. oregano
    1/2 tsp. basil
    1/2 tsp. pepper
    1/2 cup finely chopped onions
    3 cloves garlic, finely chopped
    1 cup chicken stock

Place onions, garlic and herbs in a saucepan and cover with chicken stock. Saute until onions are transparent. Add remaining ingredients and simmer over low heat, stirring occasionally for 1 1/2 hours. This sauce can be frozen or chilled until ready to use.

- **Dipping/Veggie Sauce**

    2 Tbls. mild vinegar
    1 Tbls. chick pea miso
    1 tsp. low/no sodium dijon style mustard
    2 Tbls. sesame oil

Blend vinegar, miso, mustard in a blender while slowly adding sesame oil until thickened.

- **Salad Dressing**

    1/2 cup apple cider vinegar
    1/2 cup unsweetened apple juice
    1/2 tsp. dry mustard
    1/2 tsp. paprika
    1/2 tsp. finely chopped garlic
    1/2 tsp. basil

Place ingredients in a jar, shake well and chill until ready to use.

- **No Oil French Dressing**

    2 cloves garlic
    2 med. tomatoes
    1 carrot
    1 Tbls. grated lemon rind
    1/2 tsp. basil
    1/2 tsp. paprika
    1/2 tsp. pepper
    1/2 cup unsweetened apple juice

Steam tomatoes, garlic, and carrot 3 to 5 minutes. Place in a blender with remaining ingredients and puree. Chill until ready to use.

- **Cream Dressing**

    1 medium cucumber, peeled and seeded
    1 1/2 cups low-fat yogurt
    1 Tbls. chives (fresh or frozen), chopped or 1 Tbls. scallion tops, finely chopped
    1/4 tsp. dried mint, or 1 tsp. fresh mint, chopped (optional)
    1/4 tsp. freshly ground black pepper

Puree all ingredients in a blender until smooth.

- **Lemon Dressing**

    1 cup lemon juice
    2 fertile egg yolks
    2 cloves garlic, very finely minced
    1/4 tsp. dried dill or 1 Tbls. parsley, chopped
    2 tsp. dijon mustard

Puree all ingredients in a blender until smooth.

Fruits and Desserts

• Fruit Compote

> 2 to 3 cups of any fresh, frozen unsweetened fruit
> 1/2 cup unsweetened fruit juice of choice (Heinke's fruit cider blends are nice)

Place in a saucepan and simmer until desired consistency is reached. This compote may be served hot or chilled. You may also use this as a sauce for pancakes, waffles, french toast, or to top hot cereal or rice cakes. Flavor with the following fruit/spice combinations:

> ***Blueberries***: *apple juice, ginger*
> ***Apples***: *apple juice, cinnamon, allspice, cloves, cardamon*
> ***Peaches***: *apple juice, cinnamon, ginger, apple juice and almond extract.*
> ***Apricots***: *apple juice, ginger, lemon rind, apple juice and almond extract.*
> ***Strawberries***: *pineapple juice, vanilla extract.*
> ***Raspberries***: *"Heinke's" raspberry cider and almond extract (or vanilla.*
> ***Pears***: *pear juice/apple juice, cinnamon/cardamon*

• Apple Parfait

> *2 apples, finely chopped*
> *2 tsp. cinnamon*
> *1/2 tsp. ginger*
> *16 oz. plain low/nonfat yogurt*
> *12 raw almonds, finely chopped*

Mix spices with yogurt and 1/2 almond mixture. Divide yogurt into two portions. Fold chopped apple into the first yogurt portion with almonds. Layer with balance of yogurt and sprinkle remaining almonds between each layer. Chill briefly and serve.

- **Fruit Yogurt**

    2 cups fruit of choice
    3 cups plain low/nonfat yogurt

Puree fruit in blender with yogurt and chill. Flavor with the following fruit/spice suggestions:

   Blueberry: *ginger*
   Apple: *cinnamon, allspice, cloves, cardamon*
   Peach: *cinnamon, ginger*
   Apricot: *ginger, lemon rind, cloves*
   Strawberry: *vanilla extract/almond extract*
   Raspberry: *vanilla extract/almond extract*

- **Baked Apples/Pears**

    2-4 rome or pippin apples, or pears, cored
    1/2 cup unsweetened apple juice
    1/2 tsp. cloves
    1 1/2 tsp. vanilla extract
    2 tsp. cinnamon
    1/2 cup water

Combine liquids and spices and pour over apples. Bake covered at 375 degrees for 25 to 30 minutes. Serve hot or chilled.

- **Creamy Apple Custard**

    2 cups peeled apple chunks
    2 cups apple juice
    3 Tbls. agar-agar flakes
    1 tsp. vanilla extract
    1 Tbls. tahini

Cook apples in juice until well done and then add 3 Tbls. agar-agar flakes. Cook 3 to 5 minutes stirring constantly. Remove from heat and add vanilla and tahini. Blend and refrigerate until set. Re-blend, pour into desert cups and chill thoroughly.

● Poached Pears With Raspberry Sauce

4 large bosc pears, peeled (leave stems on)
1 1/2 cups "Heinkes" raspberry cider
2 cups fresh or frozen unsweetened raspberries

Place pears and juice in a large covered saucepan and simmer 30 to 40 minutes until tender. Remove pears from juice and then reduce to 1/3 cup over high heat. Cool pan liquid and puree with raspberries in a blender.

To serve, place a small pool of raspberry sauce on a dessert place. Set pear upright on place and drizzle more raspberry sauce over the top.

● French Custard

2 fertile eggs, well beaten
1 cup R.W. Knudsen coconut nectar
1/2 Tsp. cinnamon

Blend well and pour into lightly greased baking dish. Set in water filled pan and bake at 350 degrees for 30 minutes or until a toothpick inserted into center comes out dry.

● Dates Stuffed With Almond Fudge

8 oz. jar almond butter
4 Tbls. "Hain" apple juice concentrate (syrup)
2 tsp. no alcohol, no sugar, butterscotch extract or no alcohol, no sugar, vanilla extract

Puree almond butter, apple juice concentrate, and extract until smooth. Stuff dates with almond fudge and chill. These are for special occasions only.

● **Fruit Tarts**

Crust: 1 cup oat/millet/rice flour (see recipe, page 11)
2 Tbls. sweet butter, melted
1/2 tsp. cinnamon
1 tsp. vanilla
Water as needed.

Mix well and pat into small tart pans. Prepare the filling:

1 1/2 cups sliced fruit of choice
1/2 cup unsweetened apple juice
1 Tbls. arrowroot powder
2 tsp. cinnamon
1/2 tsp. ginger

Heat juice, spices, and arrowroot until thickened and pour over fruit. Mix well and fill tart shells. Bake at 350 degrees for 25 to 30 minutes.

● **Fig Crunchies**

2 cups millet/oat/rice flour
2 tsp. cinnamon
2 fertile eggs, well beaten
1 Tsp. low sodium baking powder
2 Tbls. unsalted butter, melted
3 dried figs, finely chopped
Apple juice, unsweetened, as needed

Combine all dry ingredients. Mix in eggs, butter, and juice as needed to make a stiff cookie dough. Fold in figs and shape into walnut size balls and flatten. Place on lightly greased baking sheet and bake at 325 degrees for 15 minutes.

Variation: Used unsweetened applesauce and chopped apple instead of figs.

- **Fruit Crisp**

    3 cups sliced or coarsely chopped seasonal fresh fruit
    (apples, pears, peaches, apricots, blueberries, raspberries, etc.)
    3 Tbls. arrowroot
    1/2 cup unsweetened fruit juice of choice
    Spices of choice i.e. (cinnamon, ginger, cloves, cardamon, etc.)
    8 to 10 oz. fruit juice sweetened granola or 2 packs of your favorite natural cookies.
    1/2 cup apple juice concentrate or "Mystic Lakes" mixed fruit concentrate.

Toss fruit with arrowroot and spices of choice to evenly coat. Place in an oven proof deep dish, or a small dutch oven and pour fruit juice of choice over fruit slices.

In a blender grind granola or cookies to a fine consistency. In a bowl combine fruit concentrate and granola or cookies to form a mixture that resembles a crumb cake topping. Put this mixture on top of fruit slices to evenly cover. Bake covered at 350 degrees for 40 minutes. Remove cover and bake an additional 10 minutes. Serve hot or cold.

- **Banana Bread**

    3 very ripe bananas, mashed
    2 cups oat/millet/rice flower (see page 11)
    1 tsp. low sodium baking powder
    2 Tbls. unsalted butter, melted
    2 tsp. cinnamon
    1/2 tsp. ginger
    2 fertile eggs, or 1 yolk and 2 egg whites, well beaten
    10 raw almonds, ground into a powder
    1/2 cup plain or vanilla/pecan amasake

Combine flour with spices and baking powder. Add eggs, butter, and amasake. Mix well. Fold in bananas and nuts, pour into a lightly greased baking pan. Bake at 325 degrees for 30 to 40 minutes or until a toothpick inserted into center comes out dry.

- **Sweet Potato Pie**

    1 whole wheat pie shell
    3 cups yams, baked well and mashed
    1 Tbls. cinnamon
    1/2 tsp. allspice
    1/8 tsp. cloves
    1/8 tsp. nutmeg
    3 fertile eggs
    1 cup plain amasake

Puree together in a food processor until very smooth. Pour into pie shell and bake 1 hour at 350 degrees. Chill and serve.

- **Cream Delight Pudding**

    3 cups almond amasake or vanilla/pecan amasake
    3 Tbls. agar-agar flakes
    1/4 cup unsweetened carob chips (optional) or 1/4 cup chopped pecans (optional)

Heat amasake and agar to slow boil, stirring often until agar is dissolved. Refrigerate until set, then blend in blender. Fold in carob chips or pecans (optional) and pour into dessert cups. Chill at least 1 hour. Can be served with a garnish of carob curls using a potato peeler on a bar of unsweetened carob.

- **Fruit Gems**

    1 cup oat flour
    1/2 cup peach/apricot puree
    1/2 tsp. almond extract
    1/4 cup coconut flakes, unsweetened (optional)
    Apple juice as needed to form dough

Mix together well in a food processor to form a very stiff dough. Form into walnut size balls and chill.

● Peach Moose With Raspberry Sauce

Peach Mousse:

> *4 large ripe peaches, skinned*
> *2 1/2 cups "Heinke's" peach cider or peach juice*
> *5 to 6 Tbls. agar-agar flakes*
> *1 tsp. lemon zest*
> *1 tsp. no-sugar vanilla extract*

Cook peaches in cider until barely tender. Remove peaches from liquid and place in a blender with just enough pan juice to puree well. Add agar-agar to peach juice, bring to a boil, then reduce to simmer for 20 minutes, stirring constantly. Remove from heat and stir in vanilla, lemon zest, and peach puree. Chill until firm and re-blend in a food processor until smooth. Serve in parfait glasses topped with raspberry puree and fresh mint garnish.

Raspberry Puree:

> *2 cups fresh or frozen unsweetened raspberries*
> *1 1/2 cups "Heinke's" raspberry cider or juice.*

Reduce raspberry juice to 3/4 cup by boiling. Cool and puree well with raspberries in a blender.

● Oat Bran Muffins

> *1 fertile egg white, stiffly beaten*
> *2 Tbls. butter (raw, unsalted), melted*
> *1 1/2 cups fruit puree, apple sauce, fruit compote, or favorite similar fruit*

Mix together well and fold into:

> *1 1/2 cups oat bran*

Pour into muffin cups (lined with muffin papers) and bake at 325 degrees for 12 to 15 minutes.

● Sample Menus

Monday:

B: Oatmeal with peach compote

L: Small green salad with vinegarette dressing
Cold poached salmon with apples and limes

Snack: Fresh fruit

D: Italian chicken
Rice pilaf
Cream of cauliflower soup

Tuesday:

B: Fluffy omelette with sauted peppers and zucchini

L: Tabouli bean salad with pitas

S: Rice cakes with fruit conserves

D: Tuna in cream sauce on a bed of steamed,
Julienned zucchini

Wednesday:

B: Millet with sliced bananas and
Nonfat yogurt

L: Sliced turkey wrapped around
Steamed carrot/broccoli/yellow squash spears, spread with mustard

S: Oat bran muffin

D: Cream of celery soup
Meat loaf
Steamed swiss chard tossed with herbs of choice

Thursday

- B: Pepper or zucchini saute with rye toast
- L: Minestrone soup and eggplant/zucchini salad
- S: Fresh fruit
- D: Lamb/veal chops in balsamic sauce
  Steamed julienned carrots and green beans

Friday

- B: Five minute grain custard
- L: Soba salad
- S: Banana bread
- D: Meat ball soup
  Steamed asparagus with dijonaise sauce

Saturday

- B: No flour pancakes with apple compote
- L: Quick moo shoo veggie wraps
- S: Fresh fruit
- D: Millet pilaf
  Spicy squash
  Variety of steamed greens with butter & herbs
  Peach mousse with raspberry sauce

Sunday

- B: Van's waffles with fruit compote
- L: Nondairy zucchini quiche
  Green salad with french dressing
- S: Oat bran muffins

● *Falling Off The Wagon*

One of the most frequent calls I receive is from guilt ridden clients who have "gone off" their diets. What I like to remind them of is that health supportive eating is a flexible rather than rigid approach that actually allows for life's celebrations and indulgences as well as for the inevitable back sliding into old self comforting patterns that is part of being human.

This a natural part of the process of balancing life with lifestyle that as you come more into harmony will happen less often. What occurs after you have been applying daily Jin Shin Jyutsu® self care and choose health supportive foods a good percentage of the time, is that the foods and activities that no longer serve your well being, will simply be something you are not attracted to anymore....or if you choose them occasionally, will not impact you as much .

For those times when you have eaten widely and feel poorly afterwards, having a cup of Bieler's Soup or lightly cooked low starch veggies every few hours for 1/2 to 1 day will help a lot. If you experience weakness or have low blood sugar, just have small amounts of protein with your Bieler's / veggies.

Applying some of the Jin Shin Jyutsu® self care flows as needed from "Self Help Book" 1 will also speed your recovery. Be gentle with yourself. The process of deep change may take some time and will go easier if you focus on acceptance rather than criticism

● *Putting It All Together*

Think about selecting the easiest areas for you to integrate first, maybe picking a few ideas a month from each section to try if starting the entire program seems overwhelming. If you backslide or don't do everything "just right", know that by even making a few of the changes suggested here as part of your daily routine, you will make a huge impact on the overall quality of your life, with the bonus being a more youthful appearance.

Remember somewhere around 30 days after adding any change to your daily routines, it becomes a habit. You can then move on to implementing the next step or steps. If you incorporate 1-2 ideas a month from the entire program, in one year you will have a whole new you.

As the ancient proverb says, " A journey of a thousand miles begins with one step". Enjoy the process, be kind to yourself, and make it your own for a lifetime.

© Kaaren Jordan & Crit Taylor 2001

**website: healingessences.com
email: immune-info@healingessences.com
(805) 245-9908**

Made in the USA
Columbia, SC
04 December 2017